LGAAM

R Anatomy
Questions and Answers

First FRCR Anatomy
Questions and Answers

Usman Shaikh
Interventional Radiology Fellow, Royal Liverpool
University Hospital, Liverpool, UK

John Curtis
Consultant Radiologist, University Hospital Aintree,
Liverpool, UK

Rebecca Hanlon
Consultant Radiologist,
University Hospital Aintree, Liverpool, UK

David White
Consultant Radiologist,
University Hospital Aintree, Liverpool, UK

Andrew Dunn
Consultant Radiologist,
Royal Liverpool University Hospital, Liverpool, UK

Andrew Healey
Consultant Paediatric Interventional Radiologist,
Alder Hey Children's Hospital, Liverpool, UK

Jane Belfield
Consultant Radiologist, Royal Liverpool University Hospital, Liverpool, UK

Elizabeth Kneale
Radiology Registrar,
University Hospital Aintree, Liverpool, UK

Peter Dangerfield
University of Liverpool,
Liverpool, UK

Hilary Fewins
Consultant Radiologist,
Liverpool Heart and Chest Hospital, Liverpool, UK

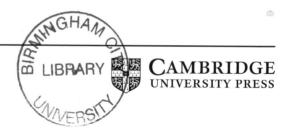

CAMBRIDGE
UNIVERSITY PRESS

CAMBRIDGE UNIVERSITY PRESS
Cambridge, New York, Melbourne, Madrid, Cape Town,
Singapore, São Paulo, Delhi, Mexico City

Cambridge University Press
The Edinburgh Building, Cambridge CB2 8RU, UK

Published in the United States of America by
Cambridge University Press, New York

www.cambridge.org
Information on this title: www.cambridge.org/9781107679498

First published 2012

Printed in the United Kingdom at the University Press, Cambridge

A catalogue record for this publication is available from the British Library

Library of Congress Cataloging-in-Publication Data

First FRCR anatomy : questions and answers / John Curtis ... [et al.].
    p. ; cm.
  Includes index.
  ISBN 978-1-107-67949-8 (Paperback)
  I. Curtis, John, 1963–
  [DNLM: 1. Anatomy–Case Reports. 2. Anatomy–Examination Questions.
3. Radiology–Case Reports. 4. Radiology–Examination Questions.   QS 18.2]
  616.07'57076–dc23

                                                        2011034134

ISBN 978-1-107-67949-8 Paperback

Contents

Foreword

Knowledge and understanding of human anatomy is a key element of medical training, whether it is at an undergraduate or at a postgraduate level. This is particularly so in interpreting radiological images. A good radiologist requires many different skills and competences, but right up there at the top of the list is a detailed knowledge of anatomy relevant to radiology. Over recent years it has become apparent that the knowledge of anatomy acquired at medical school and in specialties prior to entry to radiology training is variable and the Royal College of Radiologists has made it one of its priorities to set the standard of radiological anatomical knowledge that all radiologists should achieve. Theoretically, knowledge of anatomy should be possible to acquire as a radiology trainee passes through the modular training, but many involved in training have realized that this on its own is not sufficient. A curriculum and an appropriate form of assessment are required to ensure consistency, and there is good evidence that the need to pass an exam drives learning. The recently introduced anatomy curriculum and the First Part FRCR anatomy examination are intended to achieve this end.

Radiological images, particularly cross-sectional images, are also an excellent way of teaching anatomy to medical students, and more and more medical schools are taking advantage of this facility, as are specialties where anatomy is essential for practice within that particular area of medicine. The exciting developments in molecular and functional imaging mean that it is now even more important to be able to localize a particular function to a particular anatomical structure, and this is only possible with an excellent understanding and knowledge of anatomy.

A key element of a modern curriculum is that students should undertake regular formative assessment to allow them to evaluate their own progress and identify their training needs and that part of this should be self-assessment. There are a number of resources available to achieve this and amongst them are books produced specifically for this purpose, web-based material and the radiology – integrated training initiative (R-ITI) e-learning database (e-LD).

Dr David RM Lindsell FRCR

Preface

The reintroduction of an anatomy section heralded a welcome return to the part 1 FRCR examination. Anatomy is the main cornerstone on which radiology rests and without a good grounding, being an effective radiologist is impossible. Clinicians often call upon radiologists to guide them with anatomy in addition to steering them towards better diagnosis and management of their patients.

Our aim with this book was much more than a simple pre-examination self-assessment text. From its inception, we wanted to write a text that would prove equally as useful after the part 1 FRCR examination and therefore endeavoured to include radiological 'pearls' that would serve the radiologist well throughout his or her career. Similarly a non-radiologist reading the text would derive significant benefit in their particular field. The authors have chosen these clinical 'pearls', from within their own susbspecialties, rather than purely didactic information that might be obtained in other standard textbooks.

The cases in this book very closely match the standard type of cases likely to be encountered in the actual anatomy section of the examination.

Self-assessment gives immediate feedback to the reader which is often lacking in larger texts. Furthermore it gives a framework for further reading in the various subspecialties. We also believe that this text will be invaluable to medical students, foundation doctors and specialist trainees in surgery and medicine.

We would like to thank all of the contributing authors for their hard work in diligently putting questions together and for their shared wisdom.

Usman Shaikh
John Curtis
June 2011

Introduction

At the time of writing, the anatomy section of the part 1 FRCR examination consists of 20 digital images presented on a computer with a 19″ monitor. Each image has five questions attached, labelled a–e. You will have 75 minutes to answer a total of one-hundred questions.

The images presented are DICOM images, which have been converted into j-pegs or tiffs in order to allow annotated symbols to be applied. These images are then converted back into DICOM and uploaded onto an OsiriX database. It is *absolutely essential* to familiarize yourself with this software prior to the examination. It should be noted that the OsiriX software is only available for Apple Macs and not on IBM PCs. There is however opportunity prior to the start of the examination to manipulate sample images. The answers are to be written into a booklet.

There is further information regarding the examination available on the Royal College of Radiologists website www.rcr.ac.uk which should be part of your essential revision. There are also sample questions and answers to access.

The basics are true for any examination but need to be reiterated here.

This is not an examination to be taken lightly. The anatomy learned at medical school may be far removed from radiological anatomy in the workplace. However, more and more medical schools are using radiological anatomy to educate their undergraduates. Anatomy has been 'brought to life' in the workplace by radiologists. A good way of learning anatomy is to sit at your PACS workstation. On one screen put up a patient's chest radiograph with a CT scan of the thorax on the adjacent screen. Scrolling through the CT study allows easier explanation of the production of interfaces seen on the chest radiograph. This applies equally as well with the abdominal radiograph and CT of the abdomen and pelvis. The anatomy tested in the examination is not beyond the scope of most of the basic radiology atlases and therefore a regular consistent approach to revision is advised.

The examination is not negatively marked and therefore there must be an answer in every box.

An easy way to lose marks is not stating the side of the labelled structure, for instance, right lateral ventricle. For the purposes of this book, if there can only be one side (e.g. image of a right knee) then for ease of reading the side has not been included in the answer.

Each person has a different approach to revision and if you prefer online learning then there are a number of websites providing radiological e-learning options. Although a number of these websites are American, and therefore not geared towards the part 1 FRCR examination, there is a degree of overlap and these sites are well worth a visit. The Radiology – Integrated Training Initiative (R-ITI) should not be overlooked as it contains useful information and is written by like-minded people to who would set the anatomy examination. Other websites that our trainees have found useful include:

http://www.radiologyanatomy.com/index.php
http://www.info-radiologie.ch/index-english.php
http://www.meddean.luc.edu/lumen/MedEd/GrossAnatomy/x_sec/mainx_sec.htm
http://radiologytutorials.com/

http://web.mac.com/rlivingston/Eycleshymer/Welcome.html

http://www.rad.washington.edu/academics/academic-sections/msk/teaching-materials/radiology-anatomy-teaching-modules/

There are a number of anatomy courses now run as preparation prior to sitting the examination. Similar to mock tests in books they tutor you in key anatomy with tips to avoid simple mistakes. Their one-day format provide focussed revision and they serve as a useful adjunct.

Examination 1: Questions

Case 1.1

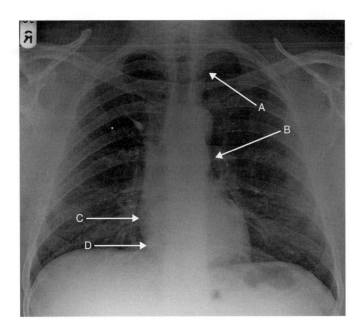

	QUESTION	WRITE YOUR ANSWER HERE
(a)	Name the structure labelled A.	
(b)	Name the structure labelled B.	
(c)	Name the structure labelled C.	
(d)	Name the structure labelled D.	
(e)	Which normal variant is present on this image?	

Case 1.2

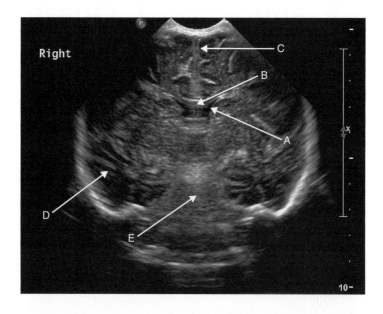

	QUESTION	WRITE YOUR ANSWER HERE
(a)	Name the structure labelled A.	
(b)	Name the structure labelled B.	
(c)	Name the structure labelled C.	
(d)	Name the structure labelled D.	
(e)	Name the structure labelled E.	

Case 1.3

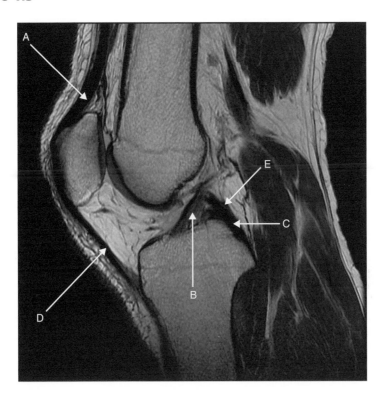

	QUESTION	WRITE YOUR ANSWER HERE
(a)	Name the structure labelled A.	
(b)	Name the structure labelled B.	
(c)	Name the structure labelled C.	
(d)	Name the structure labelled D.	
(e)	Name the structure labelled E.	

Case 1.4

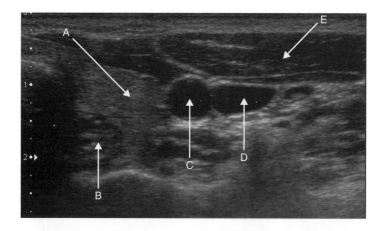

	QUESTION	WRITE YOUR ANSWER HERE
(a)	Name the structure labelled A.	
(b)	Name the structure labelled B.	
(c)	Name the structure labelled C.	
(d)	Name the structure labelled D.	
(e)	Name the structure labelled E.	

Case 1.5

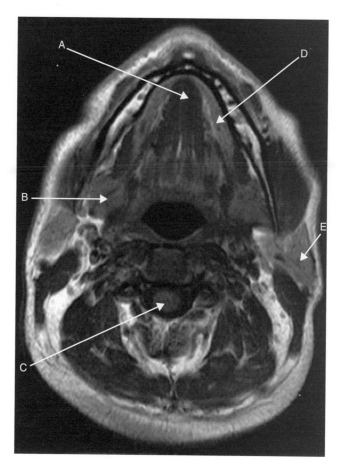

	QUESTION	WRITE YOUR ANSWER HERE
(a)	Name the structure labelled A.	
(b)	Name the structure labelled B.	
(c)	Name the structure labelled C.	
(d)	Name the structure labelled D.	
(e)	Name the structure labelled E.	

Case 1.6

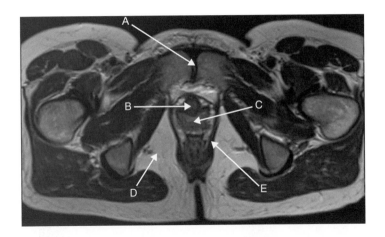

	QUESTION	WRITE YOUR ANSWER HERE
(a)	Name the structure labelled A.	
(b)	Name the structure labelled B.	
(c)	Name the structure labelled C.	
(d)	Name the vessels which run through the structure labelled D.	
(e)	Name the structure labelled E.	

Case 1.7

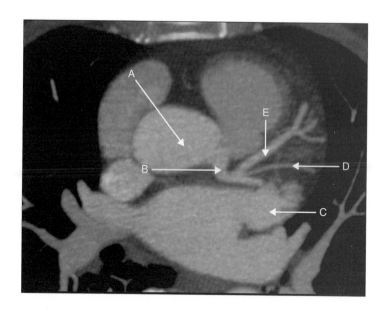

	QUESTION	WRITE YOUR ANSWER HERE
(a)	Name the structure labelled A.	
(b)	Name the structure labelled B.	
(c)	Name the structure labelled C.	
(d)	Name the structure labelled D.	
(e)	Name the structure labelled E.	

Case 1.8

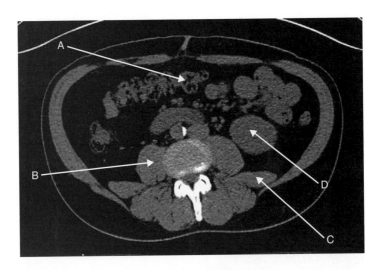

	QUESTION	WRITE YOUR ANSWER HERE
(a)	Name the structure labelled A.	
(b)	Name the structure labelled B.	
(c)	Name the structure labelled C.	
(d)	Name the structure labelled D.	
(e)	Which normal variant is present on this image?	

Case 1.9

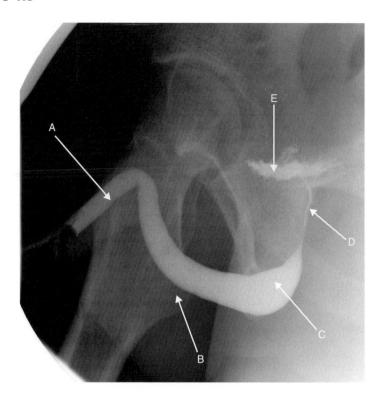

	QUESTION	WRITE YOUR ANSWER HERE
(a)	Name the structure labelled A.	
(b)	Name the structure labelled B.	
(c)	Name the structure labelled C.	
(d)	Name the structure labelled D.	
(e)	Name the structure labelled E.	

Case 1.10

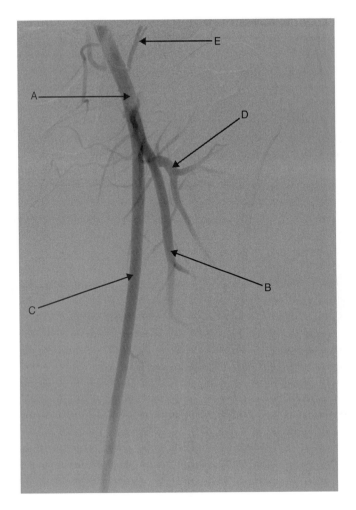

	QUESTION	WRITE YOUR ANSWER HERE
(a)	Name the structure labelled A.	
(b)	Name the structure labelled B.	
(c)	Name the structure labelled C.	
(d)	Name the structure labelled D.	
(e)	Name the structure labelled E.	

Case 1.11

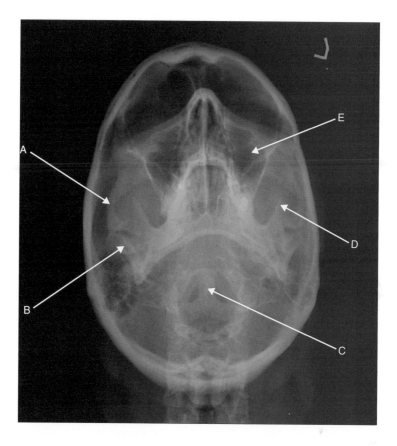

	QUESTION	WRITE YOUR ANSWER HERE
(a)	Name the structure labelled A.	
(b)	Name the structure labelled B.	
(c)	Name the structure labelled C.	
(d)	Name the structure labelled D.	
(e)	Name the structure labelled E.	

Case 1.12

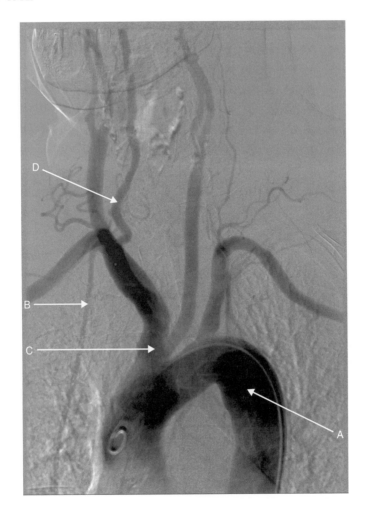

	QUESTION	WRITE YOUR ANSWER HERE
(a)	Name the structure labelled A.	
(b)	Name the structure labelled B.	
(c)	Name the structure labelled C.	
(d)	Name the structure labelled D.	
(e)	Which normal variant is present on this image?	

Case 1.13

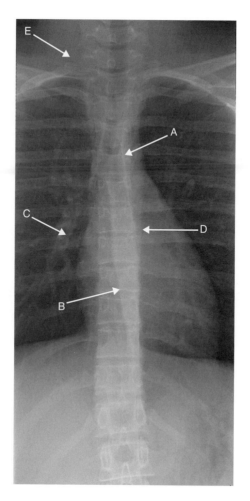

	QUESTION	WRITE YOUR ANSWER HERE
(a)	Name the structure labelled A.	
(b)	Name the structure labelled B.	
(c)	Name the structure labelled C.	
(d)	Name the structure labelled D.	
(e)	Name the structure labelled E.	

Case 1.14

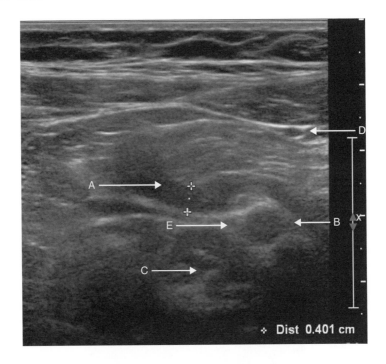

	QUESTION	WRITE YOUR ANSWER HERE
(a)	Name the structure labelled A.	
(b)	Name the structure labelled B.	
(c)	Name the structure labelled C.	
(d)	Name the structure labelled D.	
(e)	Name the structure labelled E.	

Case 1.15

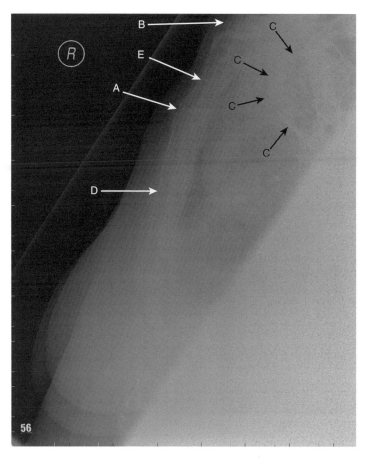

	QUESTION	WRITE YOUR ANSWER HERE
(a)	Name the structure labelled A.	
(b)	Name the structure labelled B.	
(c)	Name the structure labelled C.	
(d)	Name the structure labelled D.	
(e)	Name the structure labelled E.	

17

Case 1.16

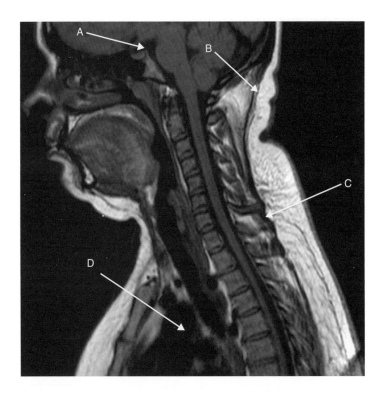

	QUESTION	WRITE YOUR ANSWER HERE
(a)	Name the structure labelled A.	
(b)	Name the structure labelled B.	
(c)	Name the structure labelled C.	
(d)	Name the structure labelled D.	
(e)	Which normal variant is present on this image?	

Case 1.17

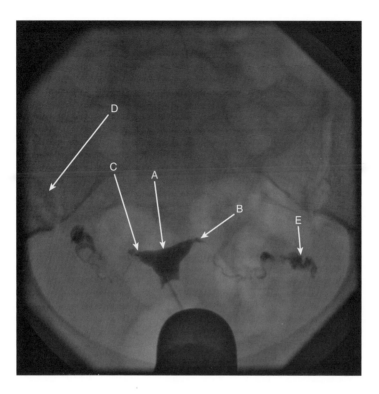

	QUESTION	WRITE YOUR ANSWER HERE
(a)	Name the structure labelled A.	
(b)	Name the structure labelled B.	
(c)	Name the structure labelled C.	
(d)	Name the structure labelled D.	
(e)	Name the structure labelled E.	

Case 1.18

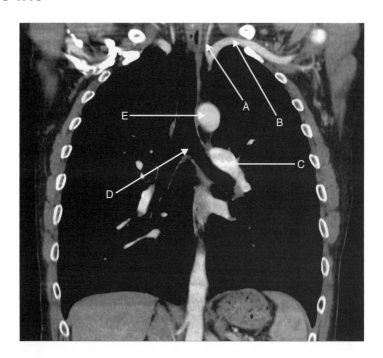

	QUESTION	WRITE YOUR ANSWER HERE
(a)	Name the structure labelled A.	
(b)	Name the structure labelled B.	
(c)	Name the structure labelled C.	
(d)	Name the structure labelled D.	
(e)	Name the structure labelled E.	

Case 1.19

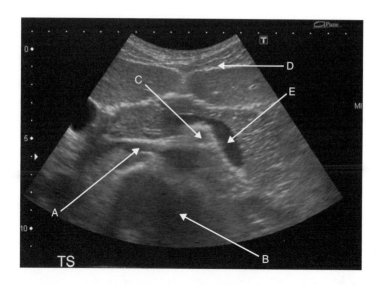

	QUESTION	WRITE YOUR ANSWER HERE
(a)	Name the structure labelled A.	
(b)	Name the structure labelled B.	
(c)	Name the structure labelled C.	
(d)	Name the structure labelled D.	
(e)	Name the structure labelled E.	

Case 1.20

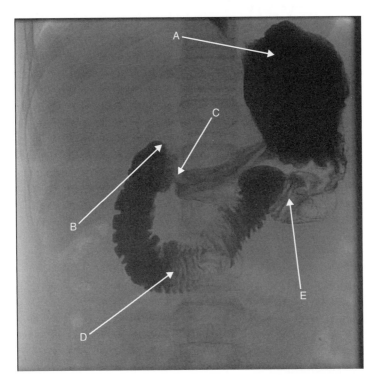

Image courtesy of Dr Alex Williams, Paediatric Radiology Fellow, Alder Hey Children's Hospital, Liverpool, UK.

	QUESTION	WRITE YOUR ANSWER HERE
(a)	Name the structure labelled A.	
(b)	Name the structure labelled B.	
(c)	Name the structure labelled C.	
(d)	Name the structure labelled D.	
(e)	Name the structure labelled E.	

Examination 1: Answers

1.1 Postero-anterior (PA) chest radiograph

(a) Left brachiocephalic vein. The left brachiocephalic vein forms a silhouette with the adjacent lung. This interface 'fades' above the clavicles as it becomes more anteriorly placed and 'merges' with the anterior chest wall.
(b) Pulmonary trunk.
(c) Right atrium (right heart border).
(d) Right cardiophrenic recess.
(e) Azygos fissure. The azygos fissure is seen in 0.5% of chest radiographs. It is formed by the caudal invagination of the azygos vein through the apex of the right upper lobe. It begins as a line in the upper portion and extends in an arc caudally toward the 'teardrop' density that is the azygos vein. The azygos vein is outside the parietal pleura – the line is therefore composed of two visceral and two parietal pleural layers. The so-called azygos 'lobe' is the segment of lung between the fissure and the trachea. It is not a true separate 'lobe' as the total bronchial anatomy in the right upper lobe has not been altered even though there may be minor variations in the bronchial supply to this segment of upper lobe.

1.2 Coronal neonatal ultrasound through the anterior fontanelle

(a) Left lateral ventricle. The combined width of the lateral ventricles on coronal imaging should be less than a third of the total width of the intracranial fossa at the same level.
(b) Corpus callosum.
(c) Superior sagittal sinus. Colour flow and Doppler can be used to assess venous sinus patency.
(d) Right temporal lobe.
(e) Pons.

Ultrasound of the neonatal brain is a very useful non-invasive diagnostic test that does not utilize ionizing radiation.
   The acoustic windows utilized include:

Anterior fontanelle until its closure at 2 years, allowing coronal and sagittal imaging of the supratentorial brain.
Posterior fontanelle up until its closure at 2 months, allowing axial imaging of the supratentorial brain.
Temporal or sphenoidal fontanelle until its closure at 3 months, allowing axial imaging of the brainstem and colour flow and Doppler of the circle of Willis.
Mastoid fontanelle allowing imaging of the posterior fossa. The mastoid process develops in the second year. The fontanelle closes towards the end of the first year.

Focal echogenic change can be related to parenchymal ischaemia or haemorrhage. Parenchymal cystic change is also well demonstrated.

1.3 Sagittal T1-weighted MR knee

(a) Quadriceps tendon. This is formed by the combination of the vastus medialis, vastus intermedius, vastus lateralis and rectus femoris tendons. Rupture of this structure results in loss of knee extension.

(b) Anterior cruciate ligament (ACL). This is an important central stabilizer of the knee joint, limiting anterior tibial translation. Failure of the ACL may occur due to tears at the origin or within the mid-substance, or less commonly following avulsion of the footprint antero-lateral to the anterior tibial spine.

(c) Posterior cruciate ligament (PCL). The PCL is a strong ligament with a recently described 4-bundle structure. Tears of this ligament most commonly occur in the mid-substance.

(d) Patellar tendon. This inserts onto the tibial tuberosity. In the clinical setting of recurrent lateral patellar dislocation, the patellar tendon insertion is surgically med-ialized by a procedure called a 'Tibial tuberosity transfer'. This reduces the degree of lateral patellar migration during knee flexion.

(e) Posterior mensico-femoral ligament (of Wrisberg). Either the posterior (Wrisberg) or anterior (Humphrey) mensico-femoral ligaments are present in 80% of knees. They stabilize the posterior horn of the lateral meniscus and must not be mistaken for displaced meniscal tear fragments on sagittal MRI images.

1.4 Transverse ultrasound of the thyroid gland

(a) Left lobe of the thyroid gland. Each lobe measures approximately 4 cm in height, and extends from the thyroid cartilage of the trachea (superiorly), to the sixth tracheal ring (inferiorly).

The recurrent laryngeal nerve runs posterior to this. This can be identified on ultrasound as a linear hypoechoic structure between the thyroid anteriorly and the longus collis muscle posteriorly.

(b) Cervical oesophagus. This lies slightly to the left of the trachea and can be confused as a mass. It is readily identified by the central echobright area representing the air and saliva in the lumen. The surrounding hypoechoic rim is muscle.

(c) Left common carotid artery. This divides into external and internal branches at the upper border of the thyroid cartilage, at approximately C4 level. The vagus nerve (cranial nerve X) runs in the carotid sheath in the infrahyoid part of the neck.

(d) Left internal jugular vein. This originates as a continuation of the sigmoid sinus and continues in the carotid sheath as it descends down the neck.

(e) Left sternocleidomastoid muscle. The muscle is a powerful rotator of the neck. Birth trauma may be associated with muscle damage, leading to contraction of the muscle causing congenital torticollis.

1.5 Axial T1-weighted MR of the salivary glands

(a) Genioglossus muscle. This large fan-shaped muscle forms the bulk of the tongue. It arises from the superior mental spine on the inner surface of the mandible and inserts along the entire length of the undersurface of the tongue. Its relaxation during sleep is thought to contribute to sleep apnoea.

(b) Right submandibular gland. This image shows an axial view through the floor of the oropharynx. The submandibular duct ('Wharton's duct') opens in the floor of the mouth on either side of the frenulum.

(c) Spinal cord.

(d) Left sublingual gland. The sublingual glands lie anterior to the submandibular gland under the tongue, beneath the mucous membrane of the floor of the mouth. Its acini secrete mucous fluid and it receives secreto-motor nerve supply from the chorda tympani nerve.

(e) Left parotid gland. The parotid glands are relatively fatty in appearance and therefore are high signal on T2-weighted and T1-weighted images.

A number of key structures run through the parotid gland including the terminal part of the external carotid artery (often giving off its two terminal branches, maxillary artery and the superficial temporal artery inside the gland), the retromandibular vein and branches of the facial (VII) nerve.

The facial nerve runs superficial to the artery and vein and divides into its five terminal branches in the gland.

Inflammation of the gland causes parotitis, often the consequence of a calculus blocking the parotid duct. Mumps may also cause painful parotitis.

1.6 Axial T1-weighted MR female pelvis

(a) Symphysis pubis. This is a cartilaginous joint between the two pubic bones whose articular surfaces are covered by hyaline cartilage. A fibrocartilaginous disc connects two surfaces allowing virtually no movement to take place.

(b) Urethra. The female urethra is usually 4 cm in length. On T2-weighted images the urethra is seen as concentric rings of different signal intensities, giving the appearance of a target.

(c) Vagina. Its lower third runs parallel to the urethra. Typically it shows an H-shaped appearance on transverse MRI. The mucosal layer shows high signal intensity on T2-weighted, muscular layer shows low signal intensity on T1-weighted and the outer adventitial layer has a high signal intensity on T2-weighted imaging.

(d) Right internal pudendal artery and veins. The structure is called the (right) ischio-anal fossa (ischio-rectal fossa). It is filled with dense fat allowing the anal canal to distend during defaecation. The pudendal nerve runs inside the pudendal canal (Alcock's canal), which is situated in the lateral wall of the ischio-anal fossa. It also contains the internal pudendal artery and veins.The inferior rectal artery, vein and inferior anal nerves also cross the fossa transversely. The ischio-anal fossa is bounded laterally by obturator internus.

(e) Left levator ani muscle. This thin muscle arises from the posterior surface of the superior ramus of the pubis and forms the medial boundary of the ischio-anal fossa. It merges with the muscle from the opposite side, the coccyx and inserts into the rectum.

1.7 CT coronary angiography

(a) Aortic root.

(b) Left main coronary artery. The left main coronary artery arises from the left coronary cusp. It bifurcates into the left anterior descending artery (LAD), which runs in the anterior inter-ventricular groove, and the left circumflex artery (LCX), which runs in the left atrio-ventricular groove.

(c) Left atrial appendage.

(d) Ramus intermedius. Occasionally (as in this case) there is a third branch from the distal left main, the ramus intermedius.

(e) Left anterior descending artery.

The LAD gives rise to diagonal branches which run over the surface of the left ventricle (LV) and also to septal perforator branches which are not well demonstrated on CT angiography (CTA). The LCX gives rise to obtuse marginal branches which run along the lateral border of the LV.

1.8 Axial unenhanced abdominal CT

(a) Transverse colon. This can be seen to cross the midline anteriorly on axial CT. It has a mesentery, the mesocolon, which attaches it to the posterior abdominal wall and on which it hangs between the fixed points of the hepatic and splenic flexures.

(b) Right psoas muscle. The psoas muscles are paired and lie lateral to the lumbar vertebrae, descending anteriorly to fuse with the iliacus muscle. A psoas abscess can develop due to the close proximity of structures to the muscle. Common origins of these abscesses include the vertebral column, expanding perinephric abscesses and bowel-related complications, such as diverticulitis.

(c) Left quadratus lumborum muscle.

(d) Left kidney. The kidneys are retroperitoneal. The hilum of the left kidney normally lies at L1 vertebral level, with the right renal hilum at the level of L1/L2 due to the liver lying superior to it. Anterior relations of the left kidney include stomach, pancreas, spleen, splenic flexure and small bowel loops.

(e) Left-sided inferior vena cava (IVC).

Normal variants are relatively common in the abdomen and include variants in vascular anatomy. Although this image is unenhanced, the IVC can be seen to lie on the left of the aorta. The aorta calcifies whereas the IVC does not, as can be seen in this image.

It is important to include any variants in vascular anatomy when constructing a radiological report as a surgeon needs to know this prior to embarking on a renal or other retroperitoneal procedures.

1.9 Urethrogram

(a) Penile urethra. The male urethra runs from the neck of the bladder to the urethral orifice at the tip of the penis. The penile and bulbous urethra constitute the anterior urethra.

(b) Lesser trochanter of the right femur.

(c) Membranous urethra.

(d) Prostatic urethra. The membranous and prostatic urethra constitute the posterior urethra.

(e) Urinary bladder (collapsed).

Urethrograms are performed by placing a small catheter in the fossa navicularis, gently inflating the balloon and slowly injecting contrast to outline the urethra. By placing the patient obliquely on the x-ray screening table this allows the penile urethra to be elongated and ensures adequate views of the entire urethra.

Proximal urethral injuries are seen with pelvic fractures as the distal prostatic and membranous urethra has a fixed attachment to the pelvic bones. It is important to perform retrograde (cystogram through suprapubic catheter) and antegrade (ascending urethrogram) studies in a patient at risk of urethral trauma to ensure there is direct continuity between the bladder and the entire urethra.

1.10 Angiogram left lower limb

(a) Left common femoral artery (CFA). This lies in the femoral sheath together with the femoral vein, which is medial to it. The femoral nerve is lateral to the sheath (mnemonic NAVY; N=nerve, A=artery, V=vein, Y=y-front). This sheath, made up of transversalis fascia anteriorly and fascia iliacus posteriorly, tapers and fuses with the vessel walls after approximately 2 cm.

The CFA is punctured at the site of maximal pulsation, usually the mid-inguinal point, halfway between the anterior superior iliac spine and pubic tubercle. While this is often described as the point of the mid-inguinal crease, it may be deceptive in old or obese patients.

(b) Left deep artery of the thigh (profunda femoris artery). This is the major arterial supply to the thigh and if the superficial artery is occluded then this vessel can supply the whole leg via collateralization to the superficial femoral artery (SFA).

A puncture too low will often result of cannulation of this vessel, increasing the risk of pseudoaneurysm formation.

(c) Left superficial femoral artery. This vessel is the main supply to the calf and foot. In patients with peripheral vascular disease this along with the iliac vessels is a common site for stenoses or occlusion. The SFA lies medial and anterior to the profunda and therefore the arterial needle should be directed that way on puncturing the CFA.

(d) Left lateral circumflex femoral artery.

(e) Left superficial circumflex iliac artery. A retrograde puncture of the CFA needs to be below this vessel to be below the inguinal ligament. This is of importance as the femoral head lies behind this segment of the CFA and therefore haemostasis can be secured by manual compression against a bony structure.

1.11 Facial bones: OM30 view (occipitomental projection with 30 degrees angulation)

(a) Temporal process of the right zygomatic bone. This meets the zygomatic process of the temporal bone to form the zygomatic arch or cheek bone. Temporalis muscle passes medial to the arch to attach at the coronoid process of the mandible.

(b) Right head of mandible. This is best seen on orthopantomogram (OPG) views or dedicated mandibular views. It articulates with the mandibular fossa of the temporal bone to form the temporomandibular joint (TMJ). These are best visualized with MR. This joint lies immediately anterior to the external auditory meatus; therefore trauma to the mandible often results with haemorrhage into the meatus which can be confused with intracerebral trauma.

(c) Odontoid peg or dens. This is part of C2 (atlas) and articulates with C1 (axis) at the atlanto-axial joint.

(d) Left coronoid process of the mandible.

(e) Left maxillary sinus. The anatomy on facial films is complex and symmetry is often useful to facilitate evaluation.

1.12 Arch aortogram

(a) Aortic arch. The ascending aorta extends to the branch of the right brachiocephalic artery and the descending aorta commences at the distal aspect of the left subclavian artery. The aortic arch lies between these two points.

(b) Right internal thoracic (or mammary) artery. This is the first branch of the subclavian artery and can act as a bypass conduit in aortic occlusion via the inferior epigastric artery. This is known as the path of Winslow.

(c) Right brachiocephalic (or innominate) artery.

(d) Right vertebral artery. This arises from the subclavian artery. The subclavian 'steal' syndrome occurs when there is a subclavian stenosis distal to the origin of the vertebral artery. The arm 'steals' its blood supply from the vertebral artery.

(e) Common origin of the left common carotid and innominate artery (bovine arch). This occurs in 22% of individuals and accounts for 73% of all arch vessel anomalies.

Other common variants include left vertebral artery arising directly from the aortic arch (6% of individuals), thyroid ima artery (6%) and aberrant right subclavian artery (1%).

1.13 PA chest radiograph centred over mediastinum

(a) Anterior junction line. This is formed by the interface of the anterior lungs as they meet in the midline. This line will only be seen on the frontal projection if there is sufficient penetration of the beam, which should be tangential to the interface. The line runs below the aortic arch and to the left in a caudal direction.

(b) Azygo-oesophageal line. This is formed by the interface between the right lung and the azygos vein and oesophagus. The cranial end of the line terminates at the point where the azygos vein drains into the superior vena cava. Any bulge of this line is indirect evidence of a possible oesophageal or posterior/middle mediastinal mass lesion and before the advent of cross-sectional imaging, this was sometimes the only plain radiograph sign of such pathology.

(c) Right interlobar pulmonary artery.

(d) Descending thoracic aorta.

(e) Right transverse process of the C7 vertebra. The transverse process of a cervical vertebra points downwards unlike that of a thoracic vertebra, which points upwards. This is a useful fact to remember when determining whether an atypical rib is a cervical or hypoplastic first rib. In the case of a cervical rib, the rib articulates with a transverse process that is pointing downwards.

1.14 Abdominal ultrasound over the right iliac fossa

(a) Appendix.

(b) Right femoral artery.

(c) Right psoas muscle.

(d) Right inferior epigastric artery.

(e) Right femoral nerve.

The normal appendix should measure less than 6 mm in its maximum diameter.
   There is often a trace of free fluid in the right iliac fossa with appendicitis.
   Careful exclusion of a faecolith should be undertaken.
   The fat surrounding the appendix should be echogenic and freely compressible.
   Colour flow Doppler signal should be the same as for the rest of the adjacent bowel.
   Enlarged mesenteric lymph nodes may be apparent and may point to the alternative diagnosis of mesenteric adenitis.
   A collection in the right iliac fossa or a pelvic collection anterior to the rectum is often appendix related.
   Compression over the inflamed appendix will result in pain and rebound tenderness can often be elicited.

1.15 Lateral radiograph of the sternum

(a) Manubrio-sternal joint (sternal angle). The manubrio-sternal joint is a secondary cartilaginous joint and may be involved with generalized seronegative arthropathies.
   Anatomically, it normally lies at the level of the T4–T5 intervertebral disc and the aortic arch.

(b) Medial clavicle.

(c) Head of humerus.

(d) Body of sternum.

(e) Manubrium.

1.16 Sagittal T1-weighted MR upper spine

(a) Optic chiasm.
(b) Nuchal ligament.
(c) Interspinous ligament.
(d) Aortic arch.
(e) Aberrant right subclavian artery. (Black spherical structure lying anterior to T2/T3.) Arterial blood flow on T1-weighted images produces a signal void. The blood vessel posterior to the oesophagus is the aberrant right subclavian artery. This is a normal variant if it is of normal calibre. When aneurysmal, this artery may cause dysphagia – the so-called *dysphagia lusoria*, which literally means 'unusual dysphagia'. An aberrant right subclavian artery causes a posterior impression on the oesophagus during a barium swallow.

1.17 Hysterosalpingogram

(a) Fundus of the uterus. This is the part of the uterus that lies above the entrance to the fallopian tubes. The body of the uterus lies below the fundus and merges with the cervix.
(b) Isthmus of the left fallopian tube. This is the narrowest part of the tube lying just lateral to the uterus.
(c) Right cornu of the uterus (uterine horn).
(d) Right sacroiliac joint. This is a synovial joint formed between the auricular surfaces of the sacrum and the iliac bones. A small but limited amount of movement occurs at this joint. An important anterior relationship is the ureter which passes over it.
(e) Ampulla of the left fallopian tube (the widest part). The uterus is almost entirely covered with peritoneum (the broad ligament) except at the anterior part of the cervix. The peritoneum reflects over the posterior wall of the bladder at the level of the internal cervical os, leaving the anterior cervix without a peritoneal covering.

The uterus is held in position within the pelvis by condensations of endopelvic fascia or ligaments that include the pubocervical, transverse cervical ligaments and the uterosacral ligaments.

1.18 Coronal enhanced CT thorax

(a) Left vertebral artery.
(b) Left subclavian artery.
(c) Left pulmonary artery.
(d) Carina.
(e) Aortic knuckle (arch).

A CT scan can be seen to be enhanced when there is contrast in the vessels. usually the thorax is scanned in the arterial phase and thereby there will be contrast in the arteries. (There will be residual denser contrast within the superior vena cava (SVC) from the venous administration.) The abdomen is commonly scanned in portal venous phase (60–70 second delay after administration of contrast), which means the portal vein will enhance more avidly compared to the arteries.

1.19 Transverse ultrasound through the porta hepatis

(a) Right renal artery.
(b) Lumbar vertebral body.
(c) Superior mesenteric artery.
(d) Left rectus abdominis muscle.
(e) Splenic vein.

1.20 Paediatric small bowel study

(a) Gastric fundus.
(b) Duodenal cap.
(c) Pylorus.
(d) Third part of duodenum.
(e) Duodeno-jejunal flexure.

This is part of an upper gastrointestinal contrast examination in an infant. The position of the duodeno-jejunal flexure (and therefore the ligament of Treitz) is crucial. It is considered normal when it meets the following two criteria: (1) it is to the left of the spine and (2) it is superior to or at the same level as the duodenal bulb.

The emphasis of this image finding is in making the diagnosis of malrotation. This occurs if *in utero* the bowel fails to rotate counterclockwise through 270 degrees, resulting in a short base of the small bowel mesentery. This can present with midgut volvulus, which requires urgent detection and intervention.

Examination 2: Questions

Case 2.1

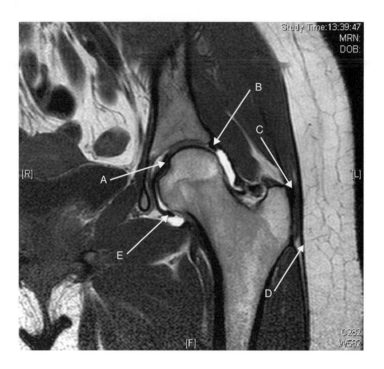

	QUESTION	WRITE YOUR ANSWER HERE
(a)	Name the structure labelled A.	
(b)	Name the structure labelled B.	
(c)	Name the structure labelled C.	
(d)	Name the structure labelled D.	
(e)	Name the structure labelled E.	

Case 2.2

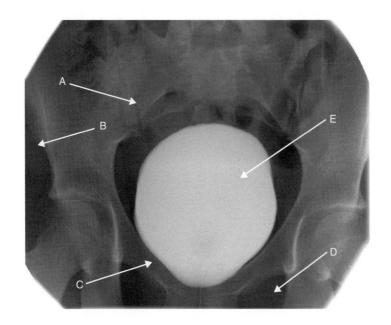

	QUESTION	WRITE YOUR ANSWER HERE
(a)	Name the structure labelled A.	
(b)	Name the structure labelled B.	
(c)	Name the structure labelled C.	
(d)	Name the structure labelled D.	
(e)	Name the structure labelled E.	

Case 2.3

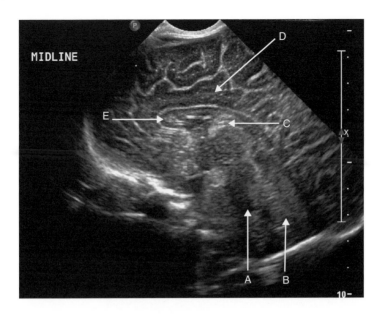

	QUESTION	WRITE YOUR ANSWER HERE
(a)	Name the structure labelled A.	
(b)	Name the structure labelled B.	
(c)	Name the structure labelled C.	
(d)	Name the structure labelled D.	
(e)	Name the structure labelled E.	

Case 2.4

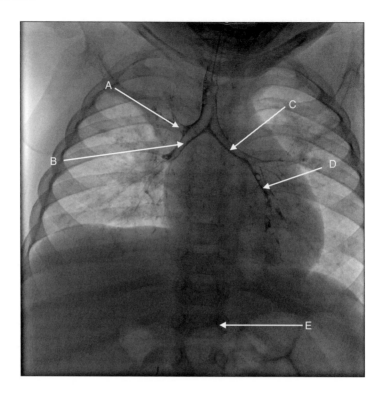

	QUESTION	WRITE YOUR ANSWER HERE
(a)	Name the structure labelled A.	
(b)	Name the structure labelled B.	
(c)	Name the structure labelled C.	
(d)	Name the structure labelled D.	
(e)	Name the structure labelled E.	

Case 2.5

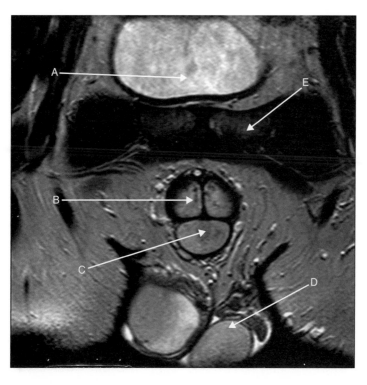

	QUESTION	WRITE YOUR ANSWER HERE
(a)	Name the structure labelled A.	
(b)	Name the structure labelled B.	
(c)	Name the structure labelled C.	
(d)	Name the structure labelled D.	
(e)	Name the structure labelled E.	

Case 2.6

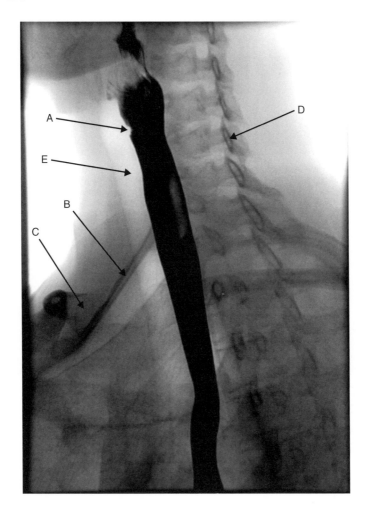

	QUESTION	WRITE YOUR ANSWER HERE
(a)	Name the structure labelled A.	
(b)	Name the structure labelled B.	
(c)	Name the structure labelled C.	
(d)	Name the structure labelled D.	
(e)	Name the structure labelled E.	

Case 2.7

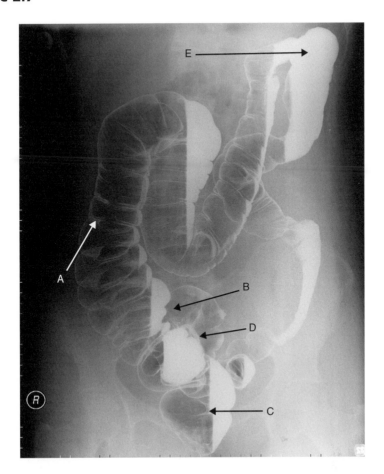

	QUESTION	WRITE YOUR ANSWER HERE
(a)	Name the structure labelled A.	
(b)	Name the structure labelled B.	
(c)	Name the structure labelled C.	
(d)	Name the structure labelled D.	
(e)	Name the structure labelled E.	

Case 2.8

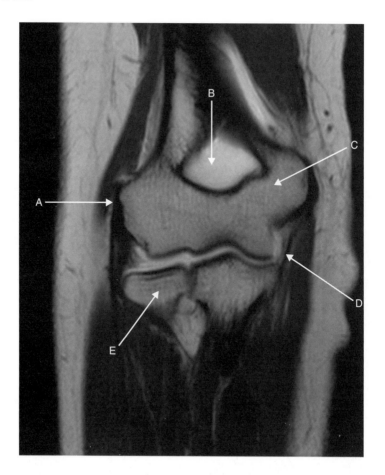

	QUESTION	WRITE YOUR ANSWER HERE
(a)	Name the structure labelled A.	
(b)	Name the structure which occupies the recess labelled B.	
(c)	Name the structure labelled C.	
(d)	Name the structure labelled D.	
(e)	Name the structure labelled E.	

Case 2.9

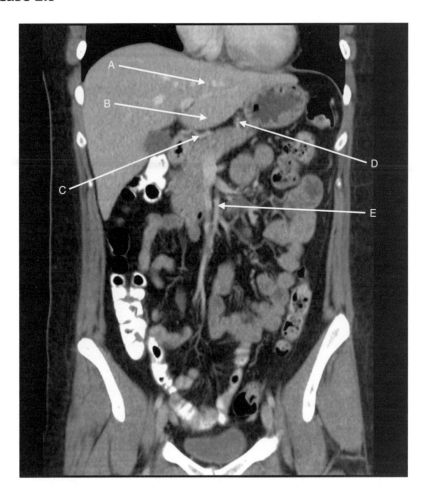

	QUESTION	WRITE YOUR ANSWER HERE
(a)	Name the segment labelled A.	
(b)	Name the segment labelled B.	
(c)	Name the structure labelled C.	
(d)	Name the structure labelled D.	
(e)	Name the structure labelled E.	

Case 2.10

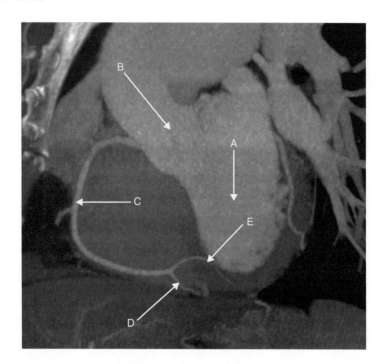

	QUESTION	WRITE YOUR ANSWER HERE
(a)	Name the structure labelled A.	
(b)	Name the structure labelled B.	
(c)	Name the structure labelled C.	
(d)	Name the structure labelled D.	
(e)	Name the structure labelled E.	

Case 2.11

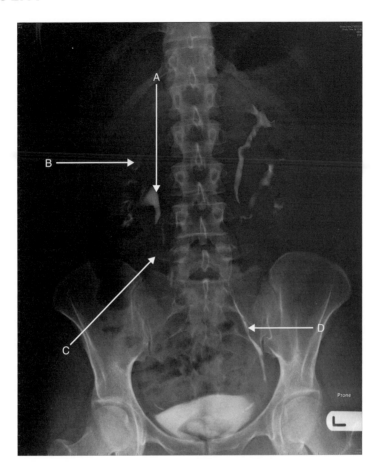

	QUESTION	WRITE YOUR ANSWER HERE
(a)	Name the structure labelled A.	
(b)	Name the structure labelled B.	
(c)	Name the structure labelled C.	
(d)	Name the structure labelled D.	
(e)	Which normal variant is present on this image?	

Case 2.12

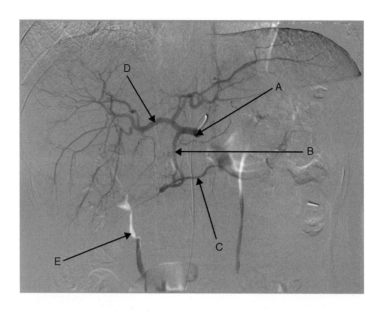

	QUESTION	WRITE YOUR ANSWER HERE
(a)	Name the structure labelled A.	
(b)	Name the structure labelled B.	
(c)	Name the structure labelled C.	
(d)	Name the structure labelled D.	
(e)	Name the structure labelled E.	

Case 2.13

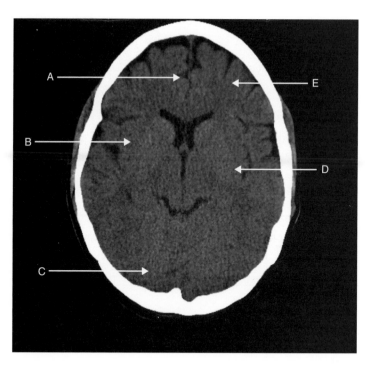

	QUESTION	WRITE YOUR ANSWER HERE
(a)	Name the artery which supplies the structure labelled A.	
(b)	Name the artery which supplies the structure labelled B.	
(c)	Name the artery which supplies the structure labelled C.	
(d)	Name the structure labelled D.	
(e)	Name the structure labelled E.	

Case 2.14

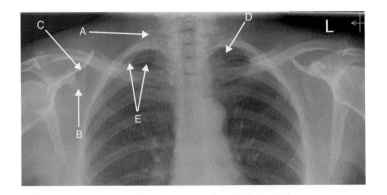

	QUESTION	WRITE YOUR ANSWER HERE
(a)	Name the structure labelled A.	
(b)	Name the structure labelled B.	
(c)	Name the structure labelled C.	
(d)	Name the structure labelled D.	
(e)	Name the structure labelled E.	

Case 2.15

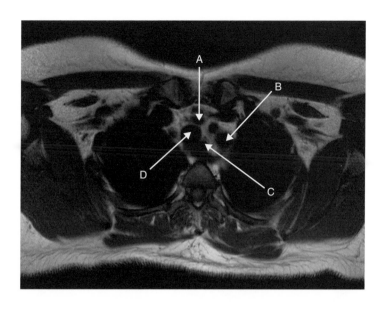

	QUESTION	WRITE YOUR ANSWER HERE
(a)	Name the structure labelled A.	
(b)	Name the structure labelled B.	
(c)	Name the structure labelled C.	
(d)	Name the structure labelled D.	
(e)	Which normal variant is present on this image?	

Case 2.16

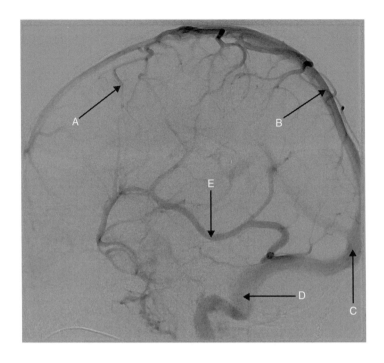

	QUESTION	WRITE YOUR ANSWER HERE
(a)	Name the structure labelled A.	
(b)	Name the structure labelled B.	
(c)	Name the structure labelled C.	
(d)	Name the structure labelled D.	
(e)	Name the structure labelled E.	

Case 2.17

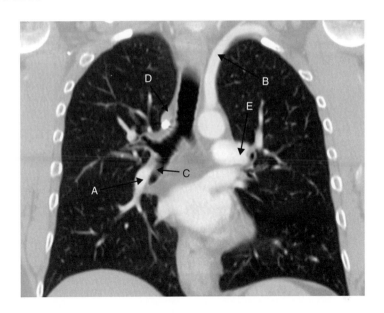

	QUESTION	WRITE YOUR ANSWER HERE
(a)	Name the structure labelled A.	
(b)	Name the structure labelled B.	
(c)	Name the structure labelled C.	
(d)	Name the structure labelled D.	
(e)	Name the structure labelled E.	

Case 2.18

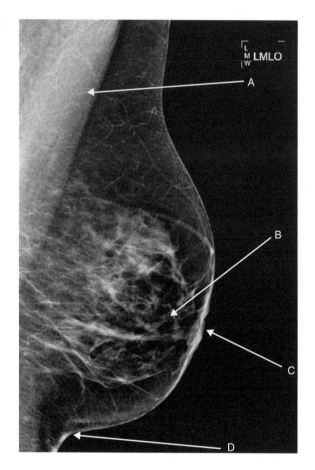

	QUESTION	WRITE YOUR ANSWER HERE
(a)	Name the structure labelled A.	
(b)	Name the structure labelled B.	
(c)	Name the structure labelled C.	
(d)	Name the structure labelled D.	
(d)	Which mammographic view has been taken?	

Case 2.19

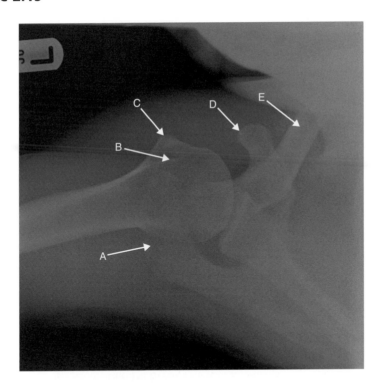

	QUESTION	WRITE YOUR ANSWER HERE
(a)	Name the structure labelled A.	
(b)	Name the structure labelled B.	
(c)	Name the structure labelled C.	
(d)	Name the structure labelled D.	
(e)	Name the structure labelled E.	

Case 2.20

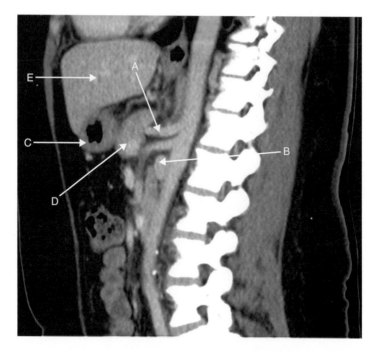

	QUESTION	WRITE YOUR ANSWER HERE
(a)	Name the structure labelled A.	
(b)	Name the structure labelled B.	
(c)	Name the structure labelled C.	
(d)	Name the structure labelled D.	
(e)	Name the structure labelled E.	

Examination 2: Answers

2.1 Coronal T1-weighted MR left hip

(a) Ligamentum teres. This strong ligament inserts into the fovea centralis of the femoral head along with important nutrient vessels.

(b) Acetabular labrum. This incomplete fibrocartilaginous ring contributes to hip joint stability. It may undergo traumatic or degenerative tearing leading to hip pain, instability and mechanical symptoms such as clicking.

(c) Gluteus medius tendon. This is an important abductor and lateral rotator of the hip that inserts upon the lateral and posterior facets of the greater trochanter.

(d) Iliotibial band (ITB) or tract. This long dense fascial band is a continuation of the tensor fascia lata muscle. It may undergo friction with resultant thickening and inflammation as it passes over the greater trochanter, producing painful, proximal ITB friction syndrome.

(e) Transverse part of the ilio-femoral ligament. The ilio-femoral ligament is a thickening of the joint capsule and is the strongest of the three hip ligaments, the other two being the ischio-femoral and pubo-femoral ligaments.

2.2 Cystogram

(a) Right sacroiliac joint.
(b) Right anterior inferior iliac spine.
(c) Right superior pubic ramus.
(d) Left obturator foramen.
(e) Contrast in bladder.

Cystograms are performed by either hand injecting, or running in a contrast infusion through either a urethral or suprapubic catheter. Both antero-posterior (AP) and lateral views should be taken, and the bladder should be filled as much as a patient can tolerate.

Bladder rupture can be either intraperitoneal or extraperitoneal. Extraperitoneal ruptures occur with fractures of the pelvis, due to the rigid fixture of the bladder neck. Intraperitoneal ruptures tend to occur in blunt trauma when the bladder is full. The tear is usually at the junction of the loose and fixed peritoneum at the posterior part of the bladder. Intraperitoneal ruptures are treated surgically, extraperitoneal ruptures are usually managed conservatively. If there is trauma, both retrograde and antegrade imaging should be performed to ensure that no ureteric trauma has occurred.

2.3 Sagittal neonatal cerebral ultrasound through the anterior fontanelle

(a) Fourth ventricle.
(b) Cerebellum.
(c) Choroid plexus.
(d) Cingulate gyrus.
(e) Corpus callosum.

The sagittal midline ultrasound of the neonatal brain allows assessment of the midline structures of the brain that are frequently affected by congenital anomalies.

The choroid plexus should be smooth in outline, uniformly echogenic and should not extend anterior to the caudo-thalamic groove. The caudo-thalamic groove is a useful landmark adjacent to the lateral ventricle where the caudate lobe and the thalamus abut each other. It is important to identify this because any echogenic structure anterior to this even if it is apparently continuous with the choroid plexus represents haemorrhage within the ventricle. An oblique sagittal scan angled through the lateral ventricle along the choroid plexus will demonstrate the caudo-thalamic groove, which can also be demonstrated scanning in the coronal plane.

2.4 Paediatric bronchogram

(a) Right upper lobe bronchus.
(b) Bronchus intermedius.
(c) Left main bronchus.
(d) Left lower lobe bronchus.
(e) Left T11 pedicle.

Bronchograms are performed in an intubated but spontaneously breathing patient to assess the patency of the large respiratory airways throughout the respiratory cycle.

In cases of bronchomalacia the airway will collapse during expiration resulting in airtrapping.

External compression of the airways or displacement related to congenital cardiac and large vessels anomalies can also be apparent.

The trachea splits into the right and left main bronchi at the carina forming a ridge between the openings of the bronchi. The right main bronchus has a shorter and more vertical course than the left; it also has a larger calibre. The right main bronchus then splits into the right upper lobe bronchus and the bronchus intermedius. The right upper lobe is divided into three segments, the apical, posterior and anterior. The bronchus intermedius divides into the short right middle lobe bronchus that supplies the two segments of the right middle lobe: the lateral and medial segments. The right lower lobe bronchus has five segmental branches: the apical, medial, anterior, lateral and posterior segments. The left main bronchus has a horizontal and long course. It divides into the left upper lobe and left lower lobe bronchi. The upper lobe bronchus supplies five segments: the apical, posterior, anterior and the two lingular segments, the superior and inferior. The left lower lobe bronchus supplies the apical, medial, anterior, lateral and posterior segments.

There are several common large airway congenital anomalies, the commonest being the pig bronchus with the right upper lobe bronchus arising directly from the trachea. They are rarely of clinical relevance unless cardiothoracic surgery is required. The pig bronchus can result in a persistently collapsed right upper lobe of the lung when the patient is intubated. This is because the tip of the endotracheal tube can be distal to the origin of the upper lobe bronchus and so can occlude it despite the tip of the endotracheal tube being in an apparent satisfactory position on plain radiographs.

2.5 Coronal T2-weighted image of the male pelvis through the base of the penis

(a) Urinary bladder.
(b) Corpus cavernosum.
(c) Corpus spongiosum.

(d) Left testis. Normal testis is high signal on T2 MRI and intermediate on T1. The epididymis is isointense or hypointense relative to testis on T1 and hypointense on T2-weighted images.

(e) Left pubic bone.

There are paired dorsal corpora cavernosa, and a single ventral corpus spongiosum, which surrounds the penile urethra. These can be seen easily on MRI or ultrasound.

Arterial supply to the penis is from the internal pudendal arteries. Paired cavernosal arteries run in the corpora cavernosa. Paired deep dorsal arteries lie external to the tunica albuginea and run laterally to the deep dorsal vein, supplying skin and glans penis.

Penile carcinoma, although relatively uncommon, can be well visualized on MRI using T2 and post-contrast T1 sequences. Primary tumours are usually solitary, ill-defined lesions that are of low signal relative to the corpora on both T1- and T2-weighted images. Tumours enhance following contrast, but to a lesser degree than the corpora cavernosa.

2.6 Barium swallow – oblique view

(a) Post cricoid venous plexus.
(b) First rib.
(c) Clavicle.
(d) Left lamina of C5.
(e) Trachea.

2.7 Left lateral decubitus film from barium enema

(a) Haustra. The muscularis propria is condensed into three narrow longitudinal bands, the taeniae coli. The taeniae shorten the colon and act as anchorage for the circular muscle. This effect causes the haustral pattern seen on barium enema.

(b) Sigmoid colon. This is entirely surrounded by peritoneum and thus has a posterior mesentery named the sigmoid mesocolon. This allows it considerable freedom of movement within the lower abdomen.

(c) Valves of Houston, or transverse folds of rectum, are formed by fusion of taeniae and support the weight of faecal matter, preventing a constant defaecation urge. They are typically less than 5 mm thick.

(d) Appendix. Its relationship to the caecum is variable. It is retrocaecal in 15% and longer than 9 cm in 25% of individuals.

(e) Splenic flexure. This is the junction between superior and inferior mesenteric arteries at the splenic flexure seen in 80% of individuals. This is the most commonly affected segment in ischaemic colitis since this region is a watershed region between the vascular territories of the inferior and superior mesenteric arteries.

2.8 Coronal T1-weighted MR elbow

(a) Common extensor origin. This is made up of the common origin of the extensor digitorum communis, extensor carpi ulnaris and extensor carpi radialis brevis tendons. Tendinopathy and partial tearing of this structure is seen with chronic microtrauma (overuse) in a condition referred to as 'tennis elbow'.

(b) Olecranon process. This is the olecranon recess, which is occupied by the olecranon process when the elbow is extended. It is a common location for intra-articular bodies which may result in a block to extension.

(c) Medial epicondyle. This bony prominence of the humerus bears the attachment of the common flexor origin. The ulnar nerve courses over its posterior surface within the ulnar tunnel.

(d) Ulnar (or medial) collateral ligament (UCL). This is an important ligament complex, composed of three bundles that act to stabilize the elbow joint and resist valgus stress. Tears of the UCL are associated with throwing sports such as cricket and baseball.

(e) Radial head. This articulates with the capitellum. Fractures of the radial head and neck are common following falls onto the outstretched arm.

2.9 Portal venous phase coronal CT abdomen

(a) Liver segment 2.

(b) Liver segment 3. The commonest classification used was first proposed by Couinaud in 1957. This partitions the liver into segments divided by the left and right branch of the portal vein and the three hepatic veins. The caudate lobe is named as segment 1.

(c) Common hepatic artery, arises from the coeliac artery into the lesser omentum ascending in front of the portal vein.

(d) Left gastric artery. This arises from the coeliac artery and passes upwards and left to reach the oesophagus. It ascends along the lesser curve of the stomach, supplying the lower third of the oesophagus and upper part of stomach.

(e) Superior mesenteric artery. This arises below the coeliac artery and descends over the uncinate process of the pancreas. It enters the root of the mesentery supplying the small intestine.

2.10 Coronary CT angiography

(a) Left ventricle.

(b) Aortic root.

(c) Right coronary artery (RCA). The RCA arises from the right coronary cusp (anterior sinus of Valsalva) and runs in the right atrio-ventricular (AV) groove. The proximal segment gives rise to a conal branch supplying the right ventricular outflow tract and a sino-atrial (SA) branch supplying the SA node in about 65% of individuals. The mid segment gives rise to an acute marginal branch supplying the right ventricle wall. The distal RCA continues in the right AV groove where a branch supplies the AV node, before continuing to the inferior surface of the heart.

(d) Posterior descending artery (PDA). In a right dominant system, the RCA supplies the PDA running in the inferior interventricular groove but in a small number individuals it is a branch of the left circumflex artery.

(e) Posterior left ventricle wall branch. This artery is a continuation of the RCA.

2.11 Intravenous urogram (IVU)

(a) Right renal pelvis.

(b) Right upper pole pyramid.

(c) L5 right transverse process.

(d) Left ureter.

(e) Left duplex kidney. This is also known as ureteric duplication, which occurs when there are two pelvicalyceal collecting systems draining one kidney. It is present in about 1% of the population and is the most common renal anomaly. If the two ureters fuse prior to entering the bladder it is called a partial duplication and is largely an incidental finding.

If the two ureters drain independently into the bladder then this becomes a complete duplication. There is an increased incidence of urinary tract infections and vesicoureteric reflux in the latter cases.

Intravenous urography has been replaced by CT urography (CTU) in many centres, but was previously an important investigation in urinary tract imaging. Contrast was injected intravenously and a series of images taken to look at function and anatomy of the renal tract. The ureters may not be completely seen due to peristalsis, and prone views can aid filling.

Remember to look at the remainder of the image for other abnormalities, including bone lesions, bowel gas pattern and any lesions seen at the lung bases.

2.12 Coeliac axis angiography

(a) Coeliac axis. This artery arises from the anterior of the aorta at a level between the T12 and L1 vertebral bodies. In 65–75% of individuals it divides into the left gastric artery, splenic and common hepatic arteries, 1–2 cm from its origin.
(b) Gastroduodenal artery. This artery lies immediately behind the first part of the duodenum and therefore ulcers in the posterior wall of the duodenal bulb can result in life-threatening haemorrhage. The first line treatment for this remains endoscopy although embolization with interventional radiology using coils or gelfoam provides a valuable alternative strategy.
(c) Superior pancreatico-duodenal artery.
(d) Right hepatic artery. The common hepatic artery arises from the coeliac axis in 75% of the population. Other common variants to be aware of include an aberrant origin of the right hepatic artery from the superior mesenteric artery (SMA) (replaced right hepatic artery in 10–12% of the population) and a replaced left hepatic artery (off the left gastric artery) in 11–12% of the population.

The blood supply to the liver is divided, with 75% supplied by the portal vein and 25% by the hepatic artery. Interestingly, however, any primary or secondary tumours in the liver invariably have an arterial supply.
(e) Right ureter.

During angiography of the gastrointestinal tract the bladder often fills with contrast and it is therefore customary and advisable to cannulate the inferior mesenteric artery first, so that views of the sigmoid colon are not obscured by an opacified bladder.

2.13 Unenhanced CT brain

(a) Right anterior cerebral artery.
(b) Right middle cerebral artery. The largest branches of the internal carotid artery (ICA) are the middle cerebral arteries, which supply the majority of the brain including the sensory and motor cortices of the head and upper limb, as well as Broca's expressive speech area.
(c) Right posterior cerebral artery.
(d) Left lentiform nucleus (part of the basal ganglia). This is a triangular area of grey matter between the internal and external capsules. Infarcts are most frequently seen in the basal ganglia which are supplied by the lenticulostriate branches from the middle cerebral artery and the resultant infarcts are called lacunar infarcts (lacuna=pond or lake. Latin).
(e) Left frontal lobe.

The vascular territories are significant if there are recent or acute infarcts in more than one territory, which imply embolic disease rather than occlusive stenosis within the carotid.

Between the vascular territories lie watershed zones where transient global hypoperfusion (cardiac arrest, general anaesthesia, systemic shock) can result in impaired flow to one or both parent vessels thereby compromising circulation to a critical level in these border zones.

2.14 PA radiograph centred over the upper chest

(a) Right first costo-transverse joint.
(b) Coracoid process of right scapula.
(c) Spine of right scapula.
(d) Tubercle of left third rib.
(e) Companion shadow of right clavicle. The companion shadow is formed by the skin and subcutaneous tissue that lies superficial to the clavicle. As the x-ray beam tangentially hits the interface between the skin and the air in the supraclavicular fossa, it produces the so-called companion shadow.

2.15 Axial T1-weighted MR of the thorax

(a) Right common carotid artery.
(b) Left subclavian artery.
(c) Oesophagus.
(d) Trachea.
(e) Aberrant right subclavian artery (ARSCA). In approximately 0.5–1% of individuals the right subclavian artery arises from the aortic arch distal to the origin of the left subclavian artery. It courses posterior to the oesophagus as it crosses obliquely to the right side. When the origin is aneurysmal (Kommerell diverticulum) it may cause dysphagia (dysphagia lusoria).

Note: in patients with a normal right subclavian artery position the brachiocephalic trunk (BCT) usually has a larger diameter than both the left common carotid and left subclavian arteries. This is because it carries arterial blood to the right common carotid and right subclavian arteries. However, in the case of an ARSCA, the artery to the right of the left common carotid artery is the right common carotid artery. This has a diameter equal to the other great vessels, unlike the BCT.

An ARSCA will cause posterior indentation of the barium column in the oesophagus during a barium swallow.

2.16 Cerebral venography

(a) Superior cerebral veins.
(b) Superior sagittal sinus. There are ten named dural venous sinuses. The brain drains centrifugally into the superficial system and centripetally towards the deep cerebral system.

Thrombus in the sinus system is diagnosed with either CT or MR; the abnormal thrombus can be discerned from the adjacent flowing blood giving rise to the 'empty delta' sign on contrast-enhanced images.

(c) Confluence of sinuses (or torcular herophili).
(d) Sigmoid sinus. These empty into the jugular vein on each side. usually the right jugular vein is more dominant and therefore larger.

The straight and superior sagittal sinuses join at the torcula to form the transverse sinus on each side which run antero-laterally to become the sigmoid sinuses.

(e) Basal vein of Rosenthal. The deep cerebral system consists most centrally of the two internal cerebral veins, which run posteriorly in the roof of the third ventricle inferior to the corpus callosum and join the basal vein of Rosenthal, as well as posterior fossa veins to form the deep cerebral vein (of Galen). This ascends for a short distance to join the inferior sagittal sinus and form the straight sinus (which are only faintly seen on this study).

2.17 Coronal CT thorax

(a) Right interlobar pulmonary artery. The right interlobar artery lies lateral to bronchus intermedius. This is useful in the recognition of these structures on a PA chest radiograph.
(b) Left subclavian artery.
(c) Bronchus intermedius.
(d) Azygos vein. Note the right paratracheal stripe which lies superior to the azygos vein.
(e) Left main pulmonary artery.

2.18 Mammogram

(a) Left pectoralis major muscle.
(b) Subareolar area.
(c) Nipple.
(d) Infra-mammary fold.
(e) Medio-lateral oblique (MLO) view of the left breast. With a properly positioned MLO view the pectoralis muscle is seen obliquely across the top of the film extending inferiorly to the level of a line drawn perpendicularly through the nipple to the muscle (the posterior nipple line). The nipple should be in profile so the subareolar tissue is adequately imaged. The infra-mammary fold should be visible so the inferior breast has been adequately imaged.

The other view utilized in breast imaging is the cranio-caudal (CC) view.

MRI of the breast has gained widespread acceptance for the purposes of breast imaging in screening, staging in primary and recurrent cancer, biopsy, treatment response and evaluating breast augmentation.

2.19 Axial radiograph of the shoulder

(a) Acromion.
(b) Intertubercular groove.
(c) Lesser tuberosity.
(d) Coracoid process.
(e) Clavicle.

2.20 CT sagittal reconstruction image of the abdominal aorta

(a) Coeliac artery.
(b) Left renal vein. The left renal vein is situated inferior to the superior mesenteric artery, anterior to the aorta.
(c) Gastric antrum. The gastric antrum is located anteriorly in contrast to the fundus, which lies more posteriorly.
(d) Head of pancreas.
(e) Left lobe of liver.

Examination 3: Questions

Case 3.1

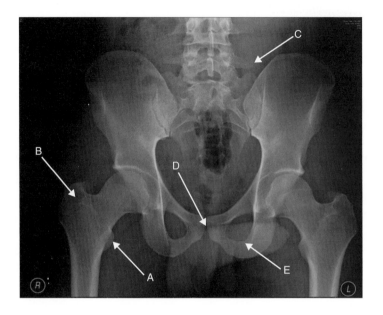

	QUESTION	WRITE YOUR ANSWER HERE
(a)	Name the structure labelled A.	
(b)	Name the structure labelled B.	
(c)	Name the structure labelled C.	
(d)	Name the type of joint labelled D.	
(e)	Name the structure labelled E.	

Case 3.2

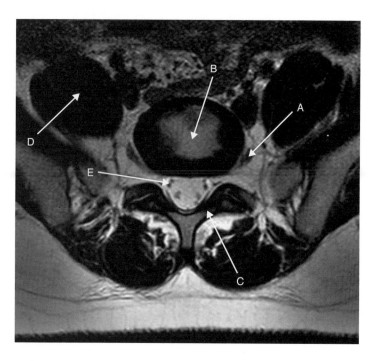

	QUESTION	WRITE YOUR ANSWER HERE
(a)	Name the structure labelled A.	
(b)	Name the structure labelled B.	
(c)	Name the structure labelled C.	
(d)	Name the structure labelled D.	
(e)	Name the structure labelled E.	

Case 3.3

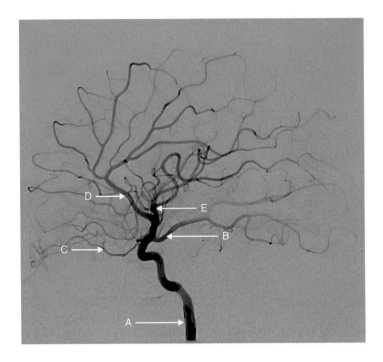

	QUESTION	WRITE YOUR ANSWER HERE
(a)	Name the structure labelled A.	
(b)	Name the structure labelled B.	
(c)	Name the structure labelled C.	
(d)	Name the structure labelled D.	
(e)	Name the structure labelled E.	

Case 3.4

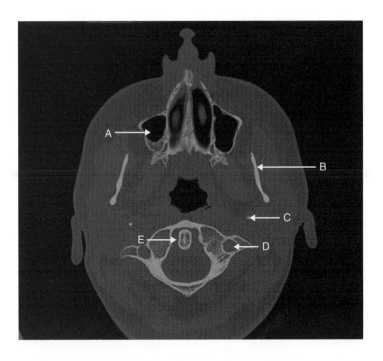

	QUESTION	WRITE YOUR ANSWER HERE
(a)	Name the structure labelled A.	
(b)	Name the structure labelled B.	
(c)	Name the structure labelled C.	
(d)	Name the structure which passes through foramen D.	
(e)	Name the structure labelled E.	

Case 3.5

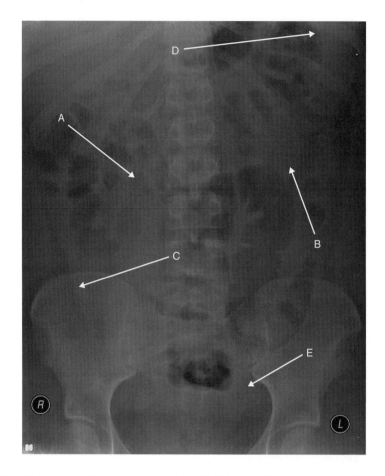

	QUESTION	WRITE YOUR ANSWER HERE
(a)	Name the structure labelled A.	
(b)	Name the structure labelled B.	
(c)	Name the structure labelled C.	
(d)	Name the structure labelled D.	
(e)	Name the structure labelled E.	

Case 3.6

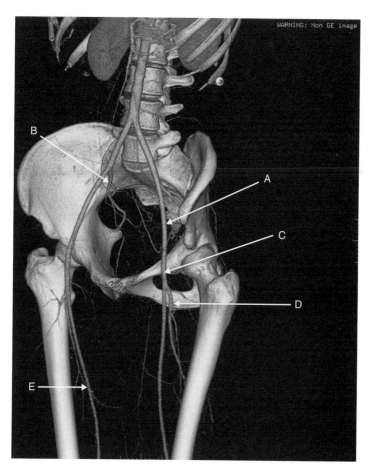

	QUESTION	WRITE YOUR ANSWER HERE
(a)	Name the structure labelled A.	
(b)	Name the structure labelled B.	
(c)	Name the structure labelled C.	
(d)	Name the structure labelled D.	
(e)	Name the structure labelled E.	

Case 3.7

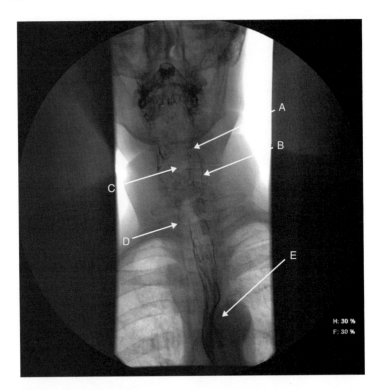

	QUESTION	WRITE YOUR ANSWER HERE
(a)	Name the structure labelled A.	
(b)	Name the structure labelled B.	
(c)	Name the structure labelled C.	
(d)	Name the structure labelled D.	
(e)	Name the structure labelled E.	

Case 3.8

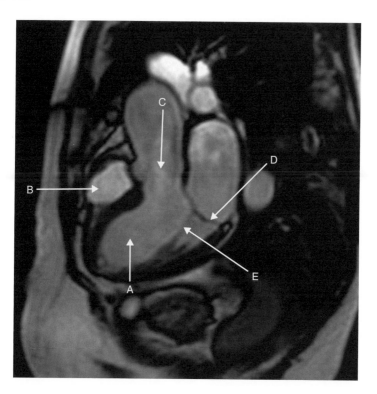

	QUESTION	WRITE YOUR ANSWER HERE
(a)	Name the structure labelled A.	
(b)	Name the structure labelled B.	
(c)	Name the structure labelled C.	
(d)	Name the structure labelled D.	
(e)	Name the structure labelled E.	

Case 3.9

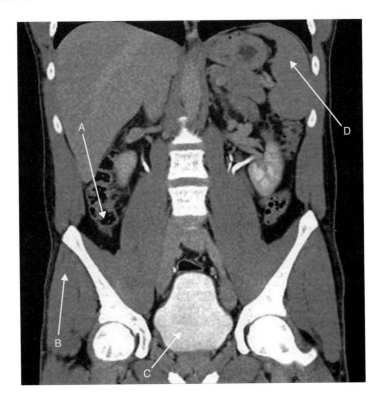

	QUESTION	WRITE YOUR ANSWER HERE
(a)	Name the structure labelled A.	
(b)	Name the structure labelled B.	
(c)	Name the structure labelled C.	
(d)	Name the structure labelled D.	
(e)	Which normal variant is present on this image?	

Case 3.10

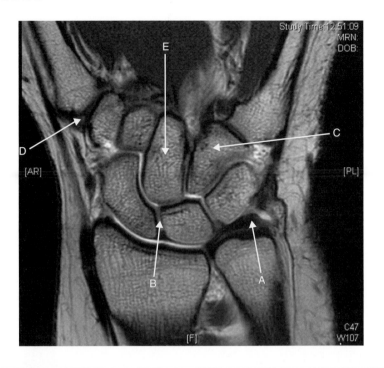

	QUESTION	WRITE YOUR ANSWER HERE
(a)	Name the structure labelled A.	
(b)	Name the structure labelled B.	
(c)	Name the structure labelled C.	
(d)	Name the structure labelled D.	
(e)	Name the structure labelled E.	

Case 3.11

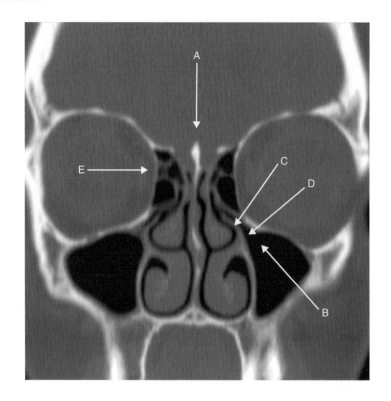

	QUESTION	WRITE YOUR ANSWER HERE
(a)	Name the structure labelled A.	
(b)	Name the structure labelled B.	
(c)	Name the structure labelled C.	
(d)	Name the structure labelled D.	
(e)	Name the structure labelled E.	

Case 3.12

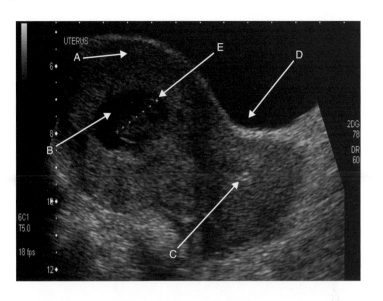

	QUESTION	WRITE YOUR ANSWER HERE
(a)	Name the structure labelled A.	
(b)	Name the structure labelled B.	
(c)	Name the structure labelled C.	
(d)	Name the structure labelled D.	
(e)	What is being measured (E)?	

Case 3.13

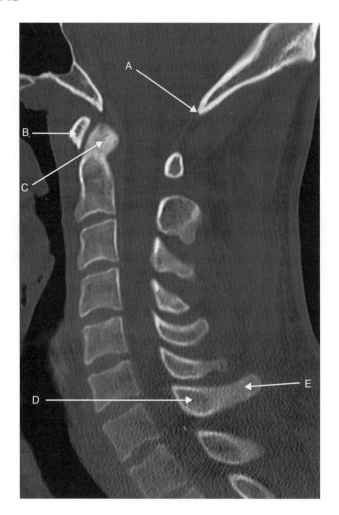

	QUESTION	WRITE YOUR ANSWER HERE
(a)	Name the structure labelled A.	
(b)	Name the structure labelled B.	
(c)	Name the structure labelled C.	
(d)	Name the structure labelled D.	
(e)	Name the structure labelled E.	

Case 3.14

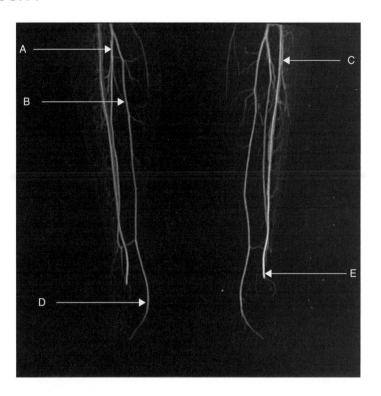

	QUESTION	WRITE YOUR ANSWER HERE
(a)	Name the structure labelled A.	
(b)	Name the structure labelled B.	
(c)	Name the structure labelled C.	
(d)	Name the structure labelled D.	
(e)	Name the structure labelled E.	

Case 3.15

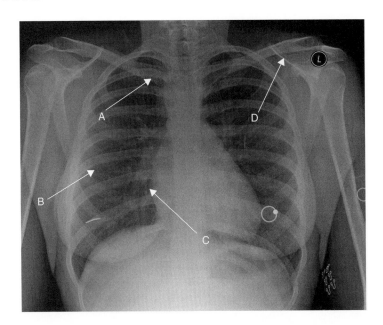

	QUESTION	WRITE YOUR ANSWER HERE
(a)	Name the structure labelled A.	
(b)	Name the structure labelled B.	
(c)	Name the structure labelled C.	
(d)	Name the structure labelled D.	
(e)	Which normal variant is present on this image?	

Case 3.16

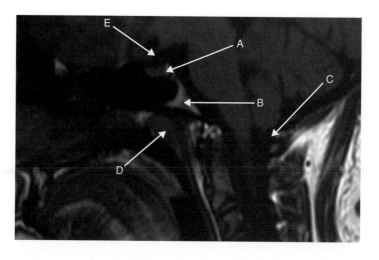

	QUESTION	WRITE YOUR ANSWER HERE
(a)	Name the structure labelled A.	
(b)	Name the structure labelled B.	
(c)	Name the structure labelled C.	
(d)	Name the structure labelled D.	
(e)	Name the structure labelled E.	

Case 3.17

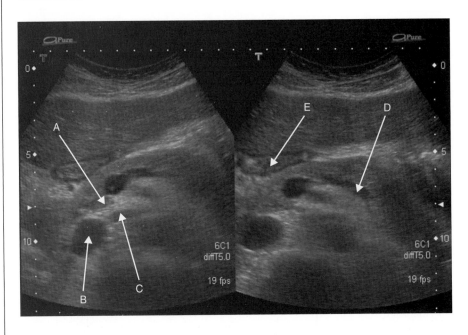

	QUESTION	WRITE YOUR ANSWER HERE
(a)	Name the structure labelled A.	
(b)	Name the structure labelled B.	
(c)	Name the structure labelled C.	
(d)	Name the structure labelled D.	
(e)	Name the structure labelled E.	

Case 3.18

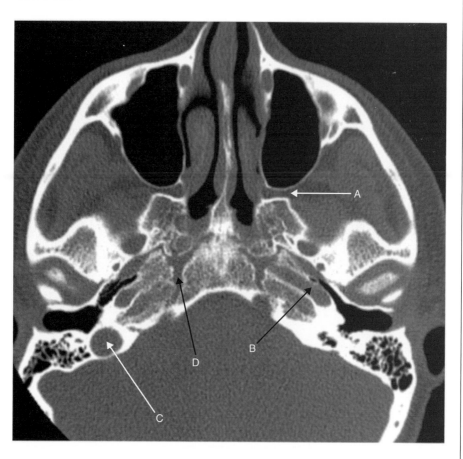

	QUESTION	WRITE YOUR ANSWER HERE
(a)	Name the structure labelled A.	
(b)	Name the nerve that runs through the structure labelled A.	
(c)	Name the structure labelled B.	
(d)	Name the structure labelled C.	
(e)	Name the structure labelled D.	

Case 3.19

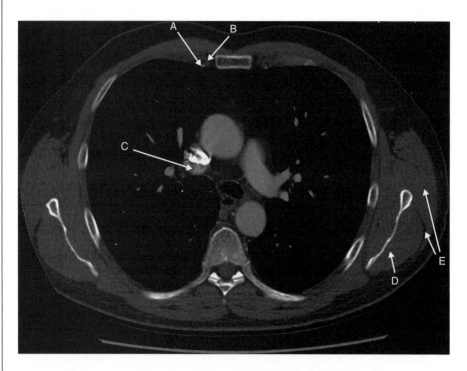

	QUESTION	WRITE YOUR ANSWER HERE
(a)	Name the structure labelled A.	
(b)	Name the structure labelled B.	
(c)	Name the structure labelled C.	
(d)	Name the structure labelled D.	
(e)	Name the structure labelled E.	

Case 3.20

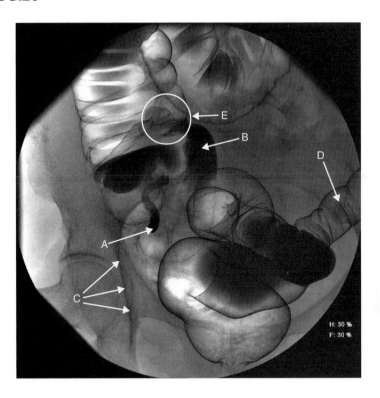

	QUESTION	WRITE YOUR ANSWER HERE
(a)	Name the structure labelled A.	
(b)	Name the structure labelled B.	
(c)	Name the structure labelled C.	
(d)	Name the structure labelled D.	
(e)	Name the structure labelled E.	

Examination 3: Answers

3.1 AP radiograph of the pelvis

(a) Lesser trochanter of the right femur. The iliopsoas tendon attaches here. This is a powerful flexor of the hip.
(b) Greater trochanter of the right femur. Gluteus medius and gluteus minimis attach here. These tendons act to perform hip abduction and lateral rotation. They can produce avulsion fractures of the greater trochanter in trauma.
(c) Left L5 transverse process. The ilio-lumbar ligament attaches here. Traction of this ligament in pelvic trauma can cause an avulsion fracture of the transverse process. It also acts as an anatomical landmark on MRI for identifying the L5 vertebral body.
(d) Pubic symphysis. It is a secondary cartilaginous joint.
(e) Left inferior pubic ramus. Adductor magnus and adductor brevis attach here acting to adduct the hip.

3.2 Axial T2-weighted lumbar spine through L5

(a) Left L5 nerve. At the level of the L5/S1 disc, the L5 nerve has already left the neural exit foramen. It may become compromised by a far lateral L5 disc herniation in this position.
(b) Nucleus pulposus of L5/S1 disc. This soft central component of the disc is surrounded by the tough outer annulus fibrosus. Annular defects result in herniation of the nucleus pulposus referred to as protrusions or extrusions, based upon their morphology. On T2-weighted images the nucleus pulposus is of high signal and the annulus fibrosus is of low signal intensity.
(c) Left lamina of L5 vertebra. Each lamina fuses in the midline to form the spinous process. The lamina is partly or completely resected (laminectomy) during lumbar disc surgery to facilitate access to the disc.
(d) Right psoas major muscle. This is a powerful hip flexor. In the clinical setting of lumbar discitis it is common to see infection tracking from the disc space into the psoas muscle to form a psoas abscess.
(e) Right S1 nerve.

3.3 Cerebral angiogram

(a) Internal carotid artery.
(b) Posterior communicating artery.
(c) Ophthalmic artery.
(d) Anterior cerebral artery.
(e) Middle cerebral artery.

There are four segments of the internal carotid artery:

1. cervical
2. petrous
3. lacerum
4. cavernous.

The circle of Willis is a ring of arteries in the suprasellar fossa that allows collateral supply to the brain. It is made up of the anterior communicating artery, anterior cerebral arteries, middle cerebral arteries, posterior communicating arteries and the posterior cerebral arteries. The circle is often susceptible to congenital anomalies and has a variable degree of completeness, demonstrating conventional anatomy in approximately one third of people.

3.4 Axial skull base CT

(a) Right maxillary sinus. The maxillary sinus is one of the paranasal sinuses. Opacification of the maxillary sinus on a plain radiograph may indicate an occult facial bone fracture following trauma; however, it can also be opacified as a consequence of other sinus diseases that result in loss of the normal sinus aeration.

(b) Left coronoid process (mandible). The coronoid process of the mandible is a site of attachment of several muscles. Temporalis muscle attaches to its internal surface and the tip while the masseter muscle is attached to the external surface.

(c) Left temporal styloid process. The styloid process of the temporal bone is a needle-like bony structure that provides the attachment sites of several ligaments and muscles:

Stylohyoid ligament

Stylomandibular ligament

Styloglossus muscle

Stylohyoid muscle

Stylopharyngeus muscle.

(d) Left vertebral artery. The vertebral artery arises from the subclavian artery and passes upwards through the vertebral foramina in the transverse process of the upper six cervical vertebra. The artery enters the skull through the foramen magnum and, at the level of the pons, the vertebral arteries from either side fuse to form the basilar artery. Within the skull the vertebral artery gives off the posterior inferior cerebellar artery and the anterior spinal artery.

The single basilar artery gives off many branches, the paired anterior inferior cerebellar arteries, multiple bilateral pontine arteries, superior cerebellar arteries. The basilar artery then bifurcates to form the posterior cerebral arteries often with one being dominant and the main supply to the occipital lobe of the brain.

(e) Odontoid peg. The odontoid peg is embryologically the body of the C1 vertebra that has fused to the body of C2 to form a prominence that facilitates rotation of the head.

3.5 AP abdominal radiograph

(a) Right psoas muscle. The psoas shadow is blurred in 19% of the population and is an insensitive sign of retroperitoneal pathology.

(b) Left kidney. The perinephric fat surrounding the kidney makes it visible.

(c) Right properitoneal fat line. This will not be visible in 18% of the population.

(d) Spleen. The outline cannot be identified in 42% of the population.

(e) Bladder outline. Like the kidneys, the distended bladder is visualized due to surrounding perivesical fat.

3.6 Volume rendering of the pelvis

(a) Left external iliac artery (not the common iliac artery as the internal iliac artery has already branched off).

(b) Right internal iliac artery.

(c) Left common femoral artery (CFA). For arterial puncture in angiogram the CFA needs to be targeted. With a puncture above (external iliac artery) or below (superficial femoral artery) this, manual compression to secure haemostasis cannot be performed adequately as the vessel cannot be compressed against bone. Furthermore, arterial closure devices are only licensed for use in the CFA.

(d) Left deep artery of the thigh (profunda femoris artery (PFA)). This artery supplies mainly the thigh while the superficial femoral artery (SFA) supplies the calf and foot. Of these the former is more important because if the SFA is occluded the calf can be supplied by collaterals from the PFA, whereas the opposite is not true.

(e) Right superficial femoral artery. This vessel is the continuation of the CFA after the deep artery of the thigh (profunda femoris artery) has branched off. At the inferior border of the femoral triangle it passes into the adductor canal (Hunter's or subsartorial canal). It emerges distally in an opening in the adductor magnus known as the adductor hiatus to become the popliteal artery.

3.7 Barium swallow

(a) Vallecula. The valleculae are paired depressions situated either side of the median glossoepiglottic fold. They separate the epiglottis from the base of the tongue and serve to hold saliva before the swallowing reflex commences.

(b) Piriform fossa. This is a recess bounded medially by the aryepiglottic fold and laterally by the thyroid cartilage. The internal branch of the superior laryngeal nerve is located immediately deep to the mucosa in this region. Fish bones can become lodged in this area.

(c) Laryngeal vestibule. This forms the opening into the larynx and is located above the vestibular folds (false cords).

(d) Air in the trachea. The trachea extends from the lower part of the larynx, level with the sixth cervical vertebra, to the upper border of the fifth thoracic vertebra. It is a midline structure but passes inferiorly to lie just to the right of midline at the level of the aortic arch (T4).

(e) Aortic arch impression.

There are three sites of natural oesophageal indentation which include the aortic arch (T4 level), the left main bronchus (T5 level) where the indentation is left-sided and the left atrium. Caustic strictures tend to occur at sites of oesophageal indentation since transit of solids and liquids is slowed at these sites.

3.8 Cardiac MR (static image from steady state free precession sequence)

(a) Left ventricle.
(b) Right ventricular outflow tract.
(c) Aortic root.
(d) Mitral valve.
(e) Papillary muscle. One of the two left ventricular papillary muscles is seen in this image. The postero-medial and antero-lateral papillary muscles are each attached to both leaflets of the mitral valve via the chordae tendinae and prevent mitral valve prolapse during ventricular systole.

This image is a single frame from a cardiac MR white blood cine (steady state free precession) examination. This 3-chamber view of the left ventricular outflow tract (LVOT) when viewed as a cine is good for visual assessment of the aortic valve and LVOT, and can also demonstrate mitral valve pathology.

3.9 Coronal enhanced abdominal CT

(a) Ascending colon.
(b) Right gluteus medius muscle.

(c) Urinary bladder.
(d) Spleen.
(e) Left duplex kidney.

CTU is now a widely accepted modality used for the investigation of haematuria. Depending on local policy, different phases of imaging are obtained, which must include a urographic phase.

Images should be interpreted using axial, sagittal and coronal planes to ensure both ureters have been adequately assessed in their entirety.

The commonest anomaly of the kidney is duplication of the collecting system, which occurs in 1% of the population. This is more common in females than males and varies from a bifid renal pelvis to complete duplication of the ureter. In this case, the ureter draining the upper pole moiety inserts lower into the bladder than that draining the lower moiety. The upper ureter is more likely to obstruct and the lower pole ureter more likely to reflux.

When evaluating CTU, look carefully for any anomaly in ureteric anatomy as one ureter may be involved in tumour or with renal calculi, and the other may be normal.

3.10 Coronal T1-weighted MR wrist

(a) Triangular fibrocartilage. This fibrocartilaginous disc contributes to stability of the distal radio-ulnar joint (DRUJ). Degenerative and traumatic tears of this structure are common causes of mechanical ulnar sided wrist pain.
(b) Scapho-lunate (SL) ligament. This short ligament is made up of volar, central and dorsal components, which contribute to stability of the proximal carpal row. Tears of the SL ligament lead to volar-flexion of the scaphoid and dorsi-flexion of the lunate producing a dorsal intercalated segment instability (DISI) appearance on lateral radiographs.
(c) Hamate. This bone occupies the distal carpal row, articulating with the fourth and fifth metacarpals. It possesses a hook-shaped process on its volar surface which bears an attachment of the flexor retinaculum. The hook may become fractured following falls onto the palm, particularly whilst holding racket handles.
(d) Carpo-metacarpal joint of the thumb. This is a synovial saddle joint which is a common site for early osteoarthrosis in the hand.
(e) Capitate. This is the largest carpal bone and the first to ossify.

3.11 Coronal CT paranasal sinuses

(a) Crista galli. This is a median ridge of bone that projects from the cribriform plate of the ethmoid bone.
(b) Left maxillary ostium. This is the opening of the maxillary sinus, located in the middle meatus of the lateral nasal cavity.
(c) Left uncinate process. This is a bony projection, formed from the medial wall of the maxillary sinus.
(d) Left infundibulum. This is the channel which drains the maxillary sinus.
(e) Right lamina papyracea. This is the paper-thin bony wall between the orbits and the ethmoid sinuses.

3.12 Fetal ultrasound

(a) Myometrium of uterus.
(b) Amniotic fluid.

(c) Endometrium of uterus.
(d) Urinary bladder.
(e) Crown–rump length (CRL).

Ultrasound is the main imaging modality used for assessment of the fetus. If there are concerns following ultrasound, MRI can be useful for further evaluation.

The role of ultrasound in the first trimester is to confirm a viable intrauterine pregnancy, determine fetal number and date the pregnancy. Nuchal thickness scanning can also be performed where increased thickness (>3 mm) is associated with chromosomal abnormalities, cardiac anomalies and skeletal dysplasia.

The CRL is measured to ascertain estimated due date. If CRL is more than or equal to 5 mm, a fetal heart beat should always be detectable. Absence of cardiac activity in embryos >5 mm is indicative of a non-viable fetus.

3.13 Sagittal CT C-spine

(a) Opisthion. This is the midpoint of the posterior aspect of the foramen magnum. Its anterior counterpoint is the basion.
(b) Anterior arch of C1 (or atlas). The C1 (atlas), C2 (axis) and C7 vertebrae are atypical.

C1 is a ring of bone with no body; the odontoid peg of C2 (dens) represents the body of C1. The articulation between C1 and C2 at the dens is called the atlanto-axial joint and is where rotation of the skull occurs. The articulation between the lateral masses of C1 and occipital condyles of the skull base is where nodding and lateral flexion occur.

(c) Odontoid peg (or dens).
(d) Posterior arch of C7.
(e) Spinous process of C7.

The C8 is a nerve root with no vertebral body. It exits the spinal canal between C7 and T1 vertebrae. Therefore, cervical roots exit above pedicles of the same numbered body. In the thoracic and lumbar spine, nerve roots exit below the pedicles of the same numbered body.

3.14 MR angiography (MRA) calf vessels

(a) Right fibular (or common peroneal) artery.
(b) Right posterior tibial artery. This artery lies deep to soleus as it runs inferiorly, becoming superficial close to the ankle joint where it it can be palpated behind the medial malleolus.
(c) Left anterior tibial artery. This is the first terminal branch of the popliteal artery. It passes forward through an opening in the intraosseus membrane and continues inferiorly. It passes anteriorly across the ankle joint beneath the extensor retinaculum to become the dorsalis pedis artery of the foot.

These three vessels (A, B and C) constitute the 'run-off' when talking about peripheral vascular disease. 'In-line flow' means at least one vessel is patent from the origin to the ankle without reliance on collateral vessels. Recent evidence suggests the longevity for below knee intervention depends upon the total number of patent vessels.

(d) Right lateral plantar artery. This together with the other branch from the dorsalis pedis, the medial plantar artery, feed into the deep plantar arch.
(e) Left dorsalis pedis artery.

3.15 PA chest radiograph

(a) Rhomboid fossa.
(b) Medial border of the right scapula.
(c) Right atrium.
(d) Spine of left scapula.
(e) Right-sided aortic arch. A right-sided aortic arch results from persistence of the right fourth branchial arch. It is more commonly seen in conjunction with an aberrant left subclavian artery. When right aortic arch is present with mirror image branching pattern (left brachiocephalic trunk, right common carotid and subclavian arteries) it is almost always associated with congenital heart disease, especially the cyanotic type.

3.16 Sagittal MR pituitary

(a) Posterior pituitary. The pituitary gland has a distinct appearance on T1-weighted sagittal MRI images. The anterior gland is isointense with white matter. The posterior pituitary signal is high because of the presence of neuropeptides in this part of the gland.
(b) Clivus. The clivus has high signal on all sequences because of bone marrow.
(c) Opisthion. This is the posterior cortical margin of the foramen magnum.
(d) Adenoidal tissue.
(e) Optic chiasm.

3.17 Transverse ultrasound upper abdomen

(a) Uncinate process of the pancreas.
(b) Inferior vena cava.
(c) Left renal vein.
(d) Splenic vein.
(e) Duodenum (D1/D2).

3.18 Axial CT skull base (bone windows)

(a) Left pterygopalatine fossa. This communicates laterally with the infratemporal fossa, and superiorly with the orbit and middle cranial fossa. Therefore, it may facilitate spread of pathology between these spaces.
(b) The maxillary division of the V cranial (trigeminal) nerve. This runs through the foramen rotundum and into the orbit via the inferior orbital fissure.
(c) Left carotid canal. This contains the internal carotid artery.
(d) Right jugular foramen. This contains the internal jugular vein, IX, X, XI cranial nerves, inferior petrosal sinus and branches of the ascending occipital and pharyngeal arteries.
(e) Right foramen lacerum. The internal carotid artery runs through its posterior aspect after emerging from the carotid canal.

3.19 Axial enhanced thorax CT

(a) Right internal thoracic (mammary) artery. The internal thoracic artery arises from the inferior subclavian artery and descends deep to the internal intercostal muscles and costal cartilages to supply the anterior chest wall and breasts, and divides at the level of the sixth intercostal space into the superior epigastric and musculophrenic arteries.

(b) Right internal thoracic (mammary) vein. This vein lies *medial* to the artery.
(c) Right main pulmonary artery.
(d) Left infraspinatus muscle.
(e) Left latissimus dorsi muscle.

3.20 Barium enema

(a) Appendix.
(b) Terminal ileum.
(c) Ilio-pectineal line.
(d) Sigmoid colon.
(e) Ileo-caecal valve.

Examination 4: Questions

Case 4.1

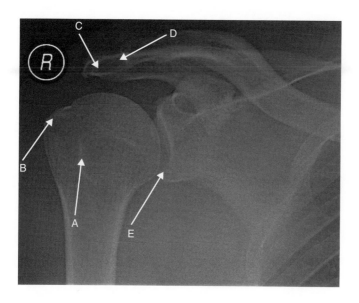

	QUESTION	WRITE YOUR ANSWER HERE
(a)	Name the structure labelled A.	
(b)	Name the structure labelled B.	
(c)	Name the structure labelled C.	
(d)	Name the structure labelled D.	
(e)	Name the structure labelled E.	

Case 4.2

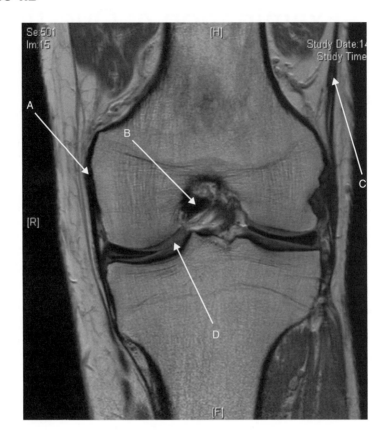

	QUESTION	WRITE YOUR ANSWER HERE
(a)	Name the structure labelled A.	
(b)	Name the structure labelled B.	
(c)	Name the structure labelled C.	
(d)	Name the structure labelled D.	
(e)	Which normal variant is present on this image?	

Case 4.3

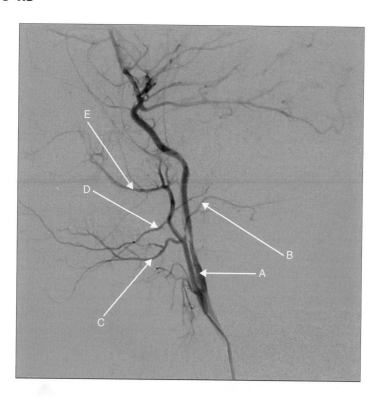

	QUESTION	WRITE YOUR ANSWER HERE
(a)	Name the structure labelled A.	
(b)	Name the structure labelled B.	
(c)	Name the structure labelled C.	
(d)	Name the structure labelled D.	
(e)	Name the structure labelled E.	

Case 4.4

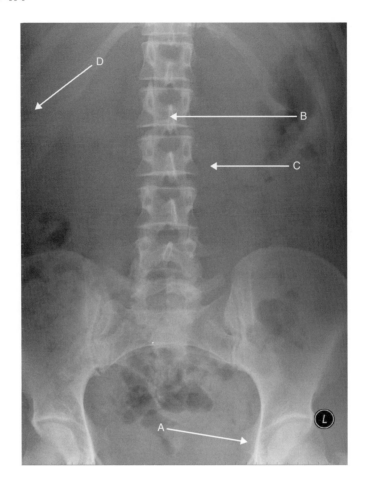

	QUESTION	WRITE YOUR ANSWER HERE
(a)	Name the structure labelled A.	
(b)	Name the structure labelled B.	
(c)	Name the structure labelled C.	
(d)	Name the structure labelled D.	
(e)	Which normal variant is present on this image?	

Case 4.5

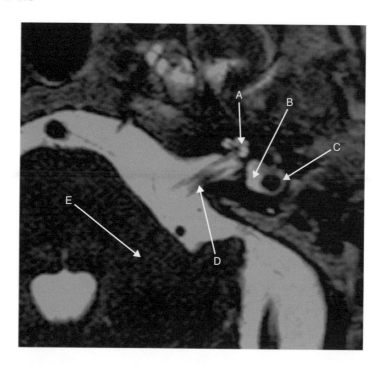

	QUESTION	WRITE YOUR ANSWER HERE
(a)	Name the structure labelled A.	
(b)	Name the structure labelled B.	
(c)	Name the structure labelled C.	
(d)	Name the structure labelled D.	
(e)	Name the structure labelled E.	

Case 4.6

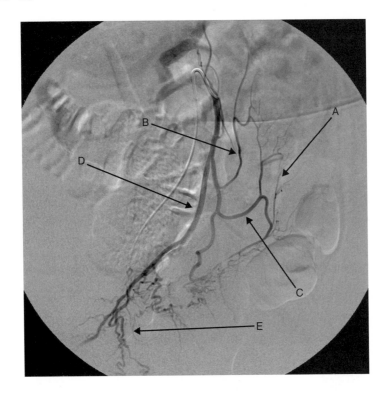

	QUESTION	WRITE YOUR ANSWER HERE
(a)	Name the structure labelled A.	
(b)	Name the structure labelled B.	
(c)	Name the structure labelled C.	
(d)	Name the structure labelled D.	
(e)	Name the structure labelled E.	

Case 4.7

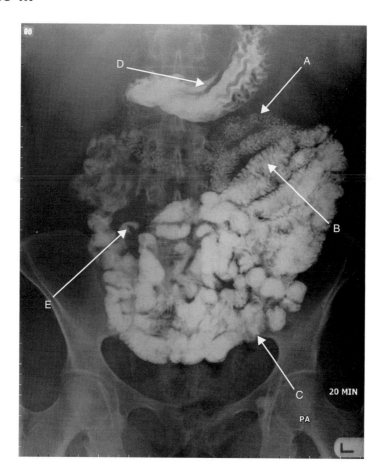

	QUESTION	WRITE YOUR ANSWER HERE
(a)	Name the structure which attaches to the point labelled A.	
(b)	Name the structure labelled B.	
(c)	Name the structure labelled C.	
(d)	Name the structure labelled D.	
(e)	Name the structure labelled E.	

Case 4.8

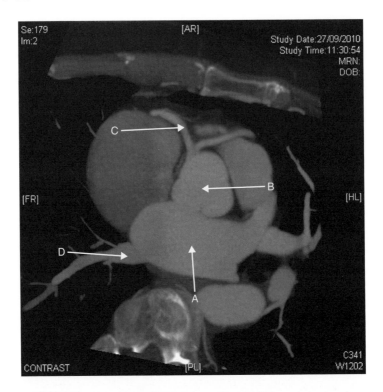

	QUESTION	WRITE YOUR ANSWER HERE
(a)	Name the structure labelled A.	
(b)	Name the structure labelled B.	
(c)	Name the structure labelled C.	
(d)	Name the structure labelled D.	
(e)	Which normal variant is present on this image?	

Case 4.9

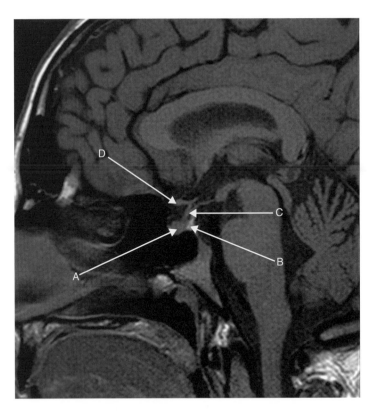

	QUESTION	WRITE YOUR ANSWER HERE
(a)	Name the structure labelled A.	
(b)	Name the structure labelled B.	
(c)	Name the structure labelled C.	
(d)	Name the structure labelled D.	
(e)	Why is the structure labelled B high signal on T1-weighted?	

Case 4.10

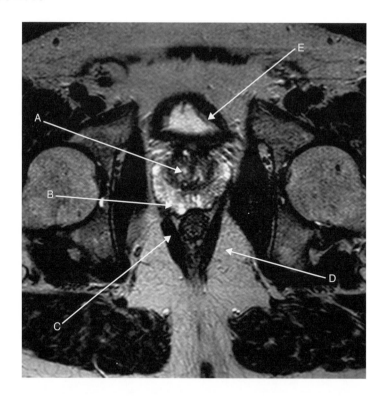

	QUESTION	WRITE YOUR ANSWER HERE
(a)	Name the structure labelled A.	
(b)	Name the structure labelled B.	
(c)	Name the structure labelled C.	
(d)	Name the structure labelled D.	
(e)	Name the structure labelled E.	

Case 4.11

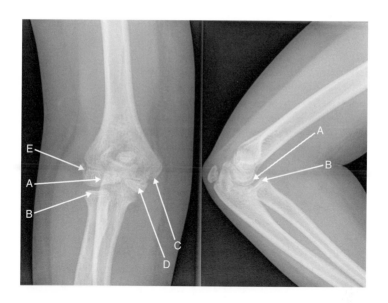

	QUESTION	WRITE YOUR ANSWER HERE
(a)	Name the structure labelled A.	
(b)	Name the structure labelled B.	
(c)	Name the structure labelled C.	
(d)	Name the structure labelled D.	
(e)	Name the structure labelled E.	

Case 4.12

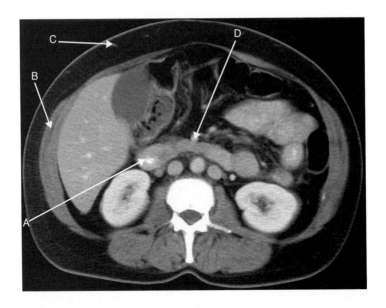

	QUESTION	WRITE YOUR ANSWER HERE
(a)	Name the structure labelled A.	
(b)	Name the structure labelled B.	
(c)	Name the structure labelled C.	
(d)	Name the structure labelled D.	
(e)	Which normal variant is present on this image?	

Case 4.13

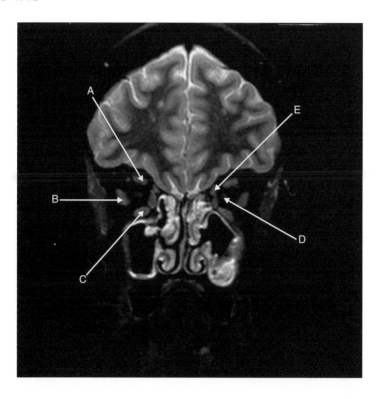

	QUESTION	WRITE YOUR ANSWER HERE
(a)	Name the structure labelled A.	
(b)	Name the structure labelled B.	
(c)	Name the structure labelled C.	
(d)	Name the structure labelled D.	
(e)	Name the structure labelled E.	

Case 4.14

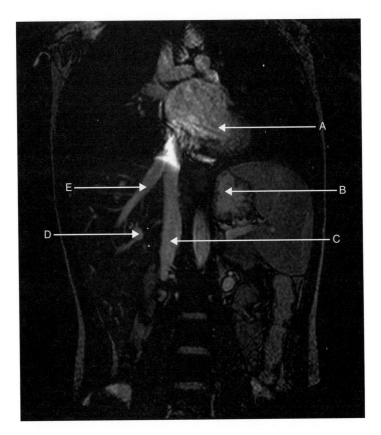

	QUESTION	WRITE YOUR ANSWER HERE
(a)	Name the structure labelled A.	
(b)	Name the structure labelled B.	
(c)	Name the structure labelled C.	
(d)	Name the structure labelled D.	
(e)	Name the structure labelled E.	

Case 4.15

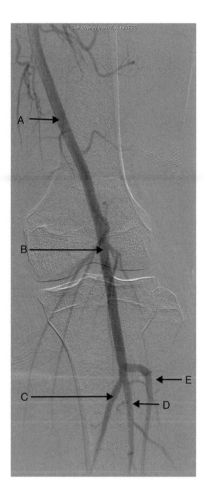

	QUESTION	WRITE YOUR ANSWER HERE
(a)	Name the structure labelled A.	
(b)	Name the structure labelled B.	
(c)	Name the structure labelled C.	
(d)	Name the structure labelled D.	
(e)	Name the structure labelled E.	

Case 4.16

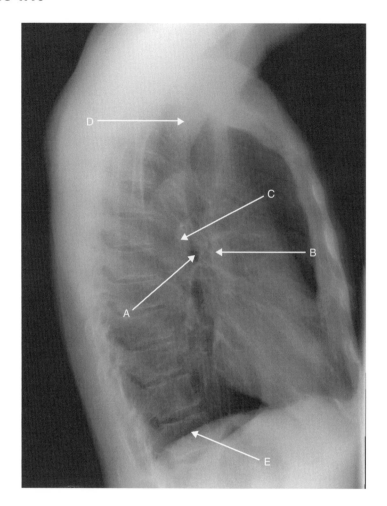

	QUESTION	WRITE YOUR ANSWER HERE
(a)	Name the structure labelled A.	
(b)	Name the structure labelled B.	
(c)	Name the structure labelled C.	
(d)	Name the structure labelled D.	
(e)	Name the structure labelled E.	

Case 4.17

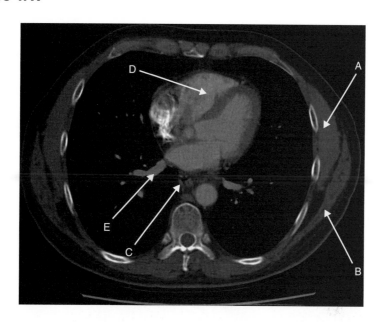

	QUESTION	WRITE YOUR ANSWER HERE
(a)	Name the structure labelled A.	
(b)	Name the structure labelled B.	
(c)	Name the structure labelled C.	
(d)	Name the structure labelled D.	
(e)	Name the structure labelled E.	

Case 4.18

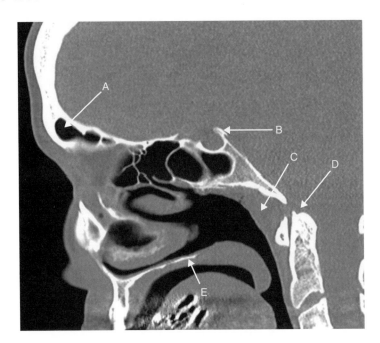

	QUESTION	WRITE YOUR ANSWER HERE
(a)	Name the structure labelled A.	
(b)	Name the structure labelled B.	
(c)	Name the structure labelled C.	
(d)	Name the structure labelled D.	
(e)	Name the structure labelled E.	

Case 4.19

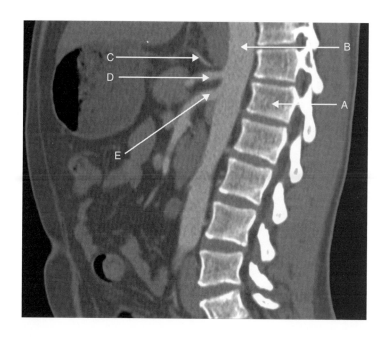

	QUESTION	WRITE YOUR ANSWER HERE
(a)	Name the structure labelled A.	
(b)	Name the structure labelled B.	
(c)	Name the structure labelled C.	
(d)	Name the structure labelled D.	
(e)	Name the structure labelled E.	

Case 4.20

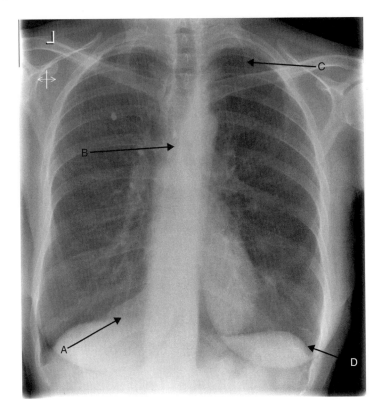

	QUESTION	WRITE YOUR ANSWER HERE
(a)	Name the structure labelled A.	
(b)	Name the structure labelled B.	
(c)	Name the structure labelled C.	
(d)	Name the structure labelled D.	
(e)	Which normal variant is present on this image?	

Examination 4: Answers

4.1 AP radiograph right shoulder

(a) Lesser tuberosity of the right humerus. The subscapularis tendon attaches here. This may rarely become avulsed during hyper-external rotation injury due to traction by the subscapularis tendon insertion.

(b) Greater tuberosity of the right humerus. This forms the bony footprint for the supraspinatus tendon.

(c) Right acromion. The coraco-acromial ligament attaches from here to the coracoid process, forming a roof over the shoulder joint. Bony enthesopathy of this ligament may contribute to subacromial impingement of the supraspinatus tendon and is implicated as a causative factor in the evolution of rotator cuff tears.

(d) Right acromio-clavicular joint. This narrow synovial joint commonly undergoes degenerative changes but may also develop erosions in inflammatory arthropathy.

(e) The antero-inferior glenoid rim. This bears the attachment of the anterior band of the inferior glenohumeral ligament, which is an important static stabilizer of the glenohumeral joint. This region may be fractured during anterior glenohumeral dislocation, producing a bony Bankart lesion.

4.2 Coronal T1-weighted MR knee

(a) Medial collateral ligament (MCL). This important ligament arises from the medial femoral condyle and inserts on the medial tibial diaphysis and resists valgus stress of the knee.

(b) Posterior cruciate ligament. This strong ligament arises from the lateral surface of the medial femoral condyle and inserts on the posterior intercondylar fossa of the tibia. It is a central stabilizer of the knee resisting posterior tibial translation.

(c) Iliotibial band (ITB). This long structure originates from the fascia of the iliotibial tract and inserts on Gerdy's tubercle on the antero-lateral tibia. Distally it may undergo repetitive friction over the lateral border of the lateral femoral condyle to produce painful distal ITB friction syndrome.

(d) Articular cartilage of medial tibial plateau. This thick layer of hyaline cartilage is composed of four zones or layers. During the evolution of osteoarthrosis the chondral layers may undergo softening, fibrillation, fissures and progressive thinning, ultimately resulting in full-thickness cartilage loss and sclerosis of the exposed sub-chondral bone.

(e) Discoid lateral meniscus. The lateral meniscus is broad, spanning the whole width of the lateral tibio-femoral compartment. This normal variant, if present, is frequently bilateral and should be examined carefully due to the high incidence of degenerative tears with this variant.

When looking at the coronal image of the knee without the fibula in view, the medial aspect is determined by the relative abundance of subcutaneous fat compared with the lateral aspect.

4.3 Cerebral angiogram common carotid artery

(a) Internal carotid artery. The internal carotid and external carotid arteries arise from the bifurcation of the common carotid artery at C4 level. The internal carotid artery gives off no branches in the neck while the external carotid artery gives off several.

Close to its origin the external carotid artery has two branches, the superior thyroid artery arises anteriorly and the ascending pharyngeal artery arises medially.

(b) Occipital artery.

(c) Lingual artery. The lingual artery is the third branch of the external carotid artery and runs anteriorly and supplies the tongue.

(d) Facial artery. The facial artery arises anteriorly, usually at the same level as the occipital artery arises posteriorly.

The posterior auricular branch is the next branch that arises posteriorly to supply the region of the pinna.

(e) Maxillary artery. The external carotid then divides to form the maxillary artery and the superficial temporal artery.

4.4 Abdomen radiograph

(a) Left ischial spine.

(b) Spinous process of L2.

(c) Left psoas muscle.

(d) Right lobe of liver (segment 7).

(e) Lumbarization of S1. This is a common congenital abnormality of the lumbosacral spine present in up to 12% of the population. The first sacral vertebra shows transition to a lumbar configuration. A more common abnormality is sacralization, where the fifth lumbar vertebra shows signs of assimilation to the sacrum.

There is no evidence to support that either abnormality predisposes to spinal pathology.

Accurate numbering of the lumbar vertebrae can be an issue in this condition and is best done counting down from the T12 vertebra.

4.5 High resolution MR through the left IAM (internal auditory meatus)

(a) Left cochlea. This is situated anteriorly within the inner ear, and consists of a spiral canal and a cone-shaped modiolus.

(b) Left vestibule. This oval chamber is approximately 5 mm in length, and contains the utricle and saccule, which form the vestibular organ responsible for maintaining balance.

(c) Left lateral semicircular canal. The semicircular canals consist of lateral, anterior and posterior divisions, which communicate with the vestibule of the bony labyrinth.

(d) Left vestibulo-cochlear nerve (VIII cranial nerve). The cochlear branch of this is involved with hearing. The vestibular branch is involved with balance and is divided into superior and inferior vestibular nerves.

The nerve lying anterior to the vestibulo-cochlear nerve is the facial nerve.

(e) Left cerebellar peduncle. The dorsal and ventral cochlear nuclei are found on the lateral surface of the inferior cerebellar peduncle.

4.6 Inferior mesenteric artery angiogram

(a) This is the arterial branch which anastomoses with the superior mesenteric artery (SMA) and is called the marginal artery (of Drummond).

(b) Ascending branch of left colic artery (or upper left colic artery).

(c) Left colic artery, middle branch.

(d) Superior rectal artery.

(e) Haemorrhoidal arteries. The inferior mesenteric artery (IMA) supplies the large intestine from the splenic flexure to the upper rectum. The proximal territory forms a watershed area with the middle colic artery and represents an area of vascular vulnerability when blood flow is reduced by any cause. This is at the splenic flexure and therefore the differential for a stricture in this lesion should include chronic ischaemia.

In the elderly there are anastomoses, arcades seen at angiography, between the SMA and IMA due to mesenteric arterial occlusion.

4.7 Barium small bowel study

(a) The suspensory ligament of the duodenum (ligament of Treitz). This is a muscle composed of a slip of skeletal muscle that arises from the proximal part of the right crus of the diaphragm as it encircles the oesophagus and inserts as a fibromuscular band of smooth muscle into the third and fourth parts of the duodenum. Contraction widens the angle of the duodeno-jejunal flexure helping the movement of bowel contents.

(b) Valvulae conniventes or circular folds (valves of Kerckring). These are reduplicated bands of mucosa that extend into the lumen of the bowel, contain a fibrovascular core of submucosa and extend completely around the whole circumference of the intestine. The folds are more crowded in the jejunum and are deeper and thicker than the ileum.

(c) Ileum. This typically makes up 60% of the small bowel and starts at 6 m.

(d) Gastric rugae. This is gastric mucosa thrown into longitudinal ridges. These are most marked towards the pyloric region and along the greater curve of the stomach.

(e) Terminal ileum. This is the most distal part of the small intestine. The terminal ileum enters the caecum obliquely at the ileo-caecal valve and partly invaginates into it. It is of paramount importance to visualize this region in small bowel studies due to the number of pathologies that occur here.

In a small bowel meal barium has been ingested by the patient and radiographs have been taken at intervals. With a small bowel enema a nasogastric tube is passed and barium introduced via this directly into the duodenum. Small bowel investigations are being replaced by MR enteroclysis, which gives similar results without the need for ionizing radiation. This is of relevance as many of these studies are carried out in young patients with inflammatory bowel disease.

4.8 CT coronary angiography

(a) Left atrium.

(b) Aortic root.

(c) Right coronary artery.

(d) Right inferior pulmonary vein.

(e) Aberrant left coronary artery. There are several normal variants of coronary artery anatomy. The illustrated example is of an aberrant left coronary artery which has a common origin with the right coronary artery from the right coronary cusp. Normally the left coronary artery arises from the left coronary cusp.

In this case the aberrant left coronary artery has a 'benign' course passing anterior to the right ventricular outflow tract (RVOT). If the aberrant artery runs a 'malignant' course between the aortic root and the RVOT this is associated with an increased incidence of sudden cardiac death.

4.9 Sagittal T1-weighted MR pituitary

(a) Adenohypophysis or anterior pituitary gland. This is five times larger than the posterior lobe, and produces hormones in response to hypothalamic releasing factors that pass down a portal venous system into the lobe.

(b) Neurohypophysis or posterior pituitary gland. This is composed of nerve fibres, extending from the supraoptic and paraventricular nuclei of the hypothalamus. Thus hormones (vasopression, oxytocin) released by the posterior pituitary are actually manufactured in the hypothalamus.

(c) Pituitary stalk. Also known as the infundibulum, this links the hypothalamus to the pituitary gland. It is composed of nerve fibres of the hypothalamohypophyseal tract and the venous portal system vessels that link the hypothalamus to the anterior pituitary.

(d) Optic chiasm. This is where the optic nerves (cranial nerve II) partially cross, and is located immediately below the hypothalamus. This is clinically important since a pituitary tumour can impinge on the chiasm leading to visual field disturbances.

(e) This is high signal because of the presence of neurosecretory granules in the neurohypophysis such as vasopressin and oxytocin. Other structures typically seen to be high signal on T1-weighted MR include:

MR contrast
melanin
fat
proteinaceous fluid
haemorrhage (due to methaemoglobin).

4.10 Axial T2-weighted MR prostate

(a) Central zone of prostate.
(b) Right peripheral zone of prostate.
(c) Right levator ani muscle.
(d) Left ischio-anal fossa.
(e) Urinary bladder.

The prostate is divided into zones:

Peripheral zone contains 70% glandular tissue
Central zone contains 25% glandular tissue
Transition zone contains 5% glandular tissue.

T2-weighted MRI images depict prostatic zonal anatomy. The peripheral zone should be seen as high signal on T2-weighted images in contrast to transitional and central zones, which are of intermediate/low signal. The transitional and central zones cannot be clearly separated with imaging.

Tumours occur in the peripheral zone where low signal lesions can be seen on T2 imaging. MRI is often performed shortly after biopsy has occurred, and it is essential to note any haemorrhagic change by carefully evaluating T1-weighted images, as this can mimic tumour. If there are difficulties in MRI interpretation due to haemorrhage and it is going to make a difference in patient management, repeat MRI may be needed. Central zone hypertrophy leads to benign prostatic hyperplasia, which can cause bladder outflow obstruction and lower urinary tract symptoms. The peripheral zone will then appear compressed on MRI, and the central zone seen to contain areas of low, intermediate and high signal.

4.11 AP and lateral radiograph left elbow

(a) Capitellum.
(b) Radial head.

(c) Medial (or internal) epicondyle.
(d) Trochlea.
(e) Lateral epicondyle.

Ossification order and times:
Capitellum – in the first year
Radial head – 5 years
Medial epicondyle – 7 years
Trochlea – 9 years
Olecranon – 11 years
Lateral epicondyle – 13 years.

While there is wide variation in ossification timing, the order of appearance of ossification is usually maintained, which therefore is more valuable to know rather than the exact dates. Sexual dimorphism should be recognized with female elbows usually ossifying and fusing earlier than males. The mnemonic CRITOL is an invaluable reminder for this order.

The ossification order assumes significance because the medial epicondyle can be avulsed and displaced into the joint. In this situation there will be an apparent well-formed trochlea with no apparent ossification of the medial epicondyle, in a child younger than 9 years. In an older child there may appear to be a fragmented or bifid trochlea, but no medial epicondyle. There may be other clues to a significant injury being present including soft tissue swelling or a joint effusion. However, soft tissue swelling may be minimal as this injury is often an avulsion injury and not direct trauma. A joint effusion may not be present if there is disruption of the joint capsule allowing the effusion to escape into the soft tissues without raising the anterior and posterior fat pads that are usually apparent with elbow joint effusions. In some cases CT or MRI assessment may be required to confirm or exclude injury.

4.12 Axial portal venous phase abdominal CT

(a) Duodenum – second part.
(b) Right external oblique muscle.
(c) Right inferior epigastric artery.
(d) Superior mesenteric artery.
(e) Left-sided component of a duplicated inferior vena cava (IVC).

A double IVC has a prevalence of up to 3% and comprises a right- and left-sided IVC, which occur below the level of the renal veins. The two cavae join when the left-sided component crosses the midline, usually anterior to the aorta to join the left renal vein, which drains into the right-sided IVC. Occasionally the right renal vein may be retro-aortic.

A left-sided infra-renal IVC is described, having a prevalence of up to 0.5%. As it ascends, it crosses the midline anterior to the aorta as it joins the left renal vein.

The most important clinical problem in both anomalies is a tendency for misdiagnosis as left para-aortic lymphadenopathy. It can rarely assume relevance in IVC filter placement in which case bilateral iliac filters can be considered.

4.13 Coronal MR brain: orbital muscles

(a) Right superior rectus muscle.
(b) Right lateral rectus muscle.
(c) Right inferior rectus muscle.

(d) Left optic nerve.

(e) Left superior oblique muscle.

There are six extrinsic ocular muscles that insert into the sclera: four rectus muscles (superior, inferior, medial and lateral recti), the superior oblique and inferior oblique. These can be visualized on CT or MRI.

Ocular muscles may be affected in thyroid eye disease, in one or both orbits. The inferior and medial rectus muscles are more likely to be involved first (mnemonic that gives the order of extraocular muscle involvement – I'M SLow – inferior, medial, superior, lateral). Swelling occurs involving the belly of the muscles but sparing of the tendon, whereas in orbital pseudotumour or myositis, the anterior tendinous portion is also involved.

Note the presence of mucosal thickening in the maxillary sinuses.

4.14 Coronal T2-weighted MR through thorax and abdomen

(a) Left ventricle.

(b) Fundus of stomach.

(c) Inferior vena cava (IVC). The IVC passes through the central tendon of the diaphragm at T8 together with the right phrenic nerve. The oesophagus passes through the diaphragm at T10 together with the right vagus nerve posteriorly and the left vagus nerve anteriorly. The aortic opening is at T12 through which also passes the thoracic duct. Other structures which pass through the diaphragm are the left phrenic nerve, splanchnic nerves and the sympathetic chain behind the arcuate ligaments.

(d) Right portal vein. The proximity of the portal vein to the hepatic vein allows for a Transjugular Intrahepatic Porto-systemic Shunt (or TIPSS) procedure. With cirrhosis of the liver there is raised venous pressure in the liver bed which transmits to the portal circulation and collateral pathways develop. In particular, there is risk of catastrophic gastrointestinal haemorrhage from oesophogeal varices. A TIPSS procedure shunts blood into the systemic circulation thereby reducing portal pressure. It involves placing a covered stent between the right portal vein and right hepatic vein via a jugular approach.

(e) Right hepatic vein.

4.15 Angiogram left lower limb

(a) Superficial femoral artery. Distally this lies in the adductor canal lying on adductor longus, then adductor magnus, becoming the popliteal artery as it passes through the adductor hiatus in latter muscle.

(b) Popliteal artery. The popliteal artery branches into its end arteries at the lower border of popliteus in 95% of individuals. However, in particular, there is variability in the level of branching of the anterior tibial artery.

(c) Posterior tibial (PT) artery. The segment of vessel between the popliteal artery and bifurcation of the PT and peroneal artery is referred to as the tibio-peroneal trunk.

(d) Fibular (common peroneal) artery. Normally the fibular (peroneal) artery terminates in the distal calf.

(e) Anterior tibial artery. The anterior and posterior tibial arteries continue into the foot as the dorsalis pedis and lateral plantar arteries respectively.

4.16 Lateral chest radiograph

(a) Left main bronchus.

(b) Right pulmonary artery.

(c) Left pulmonary artery. The left pulmonary artery is *posterior* to the right pulmonary artery on the lateral projection and lies superior to the relatively horizontally orientated left main bronchus, which appears as an oval lucency (A).

(d) Posterior tracheal stripe. The posterior tracheal stripe should be no greater than 2.5 mm in thickness when the posterior tracheal wall coming into contact with the upper lobe forms the stripe. The posterior tracheal stripe will be up to 5.5 mm thickness if there is apposition of the anterior oesophageal wall and the posterior trachea.

Raider's (retrotracheal) triangle is bounded by the thoracic inlet superiorly, aortic arch inferiorly, the spine posteriorly and the posterior tracheal stripe anteriorly.

(e) Left hemidiaphragm. Determining the side of the hemidiaphragm on the lateral film is reasonably straightforward. The diaphragm that is 'lost' under the cardiac silhouette is the left hemidiaphragm because it has the same radiographic density as the heart. If the gastric bubble is above one hemidiaphragm and below another, then it is below the left hemidiaphragm (if the gastric bubble is below both hemidiaphragms, this method cannot be used to determine the side).

4.17 Axial enhanced CT thorax

(a) Left serratus anterior muscle.
(b) Left latissimus dorsi muscle.
(c) Oesophagus.
(d) Right ventricle.
(e) Right inferior pulmonary vein.

The pulmonary veins enter the left atrium almost perpendicular to the lateral atrial walls. The inferior and superior pulmonary veins enter the atrium very close to each other.

Pulmonary veins run in the interlobular septa along with lymphatics. They enter the left atrium at the hilum and may enter the atrium separately – one for each lobe – or may conjoin before entering the atrium.

Pulmonary veins lie *anterior* to pulmonary arteries bilaterally.

4.18 Sagittal paranasal sinuses

(a) Frontal sinus.
(b) Dorsum sellae.
(c) Adenoidal tissue.
(d) Cruciate ligament of atlas.
(e) Hard palate.

4.19 Sagittal minimal intensity projection (MIP) abdominal aorta

(a) T12 vertebral body.
(b) Aorta.
(c) Left gastric artery.
(d) Coeliac axis.
(e) Superior mesenteric artery (SMA). The SMA comes off at L1, which is known as the transpyloric plane of Addison. Its usefulness is in the number of structures which lie in this plane:
Pylorus of stomach
Fundus of gallbladder

Neck of pancreas
Renal pelvis
Termination of spinal cord
Ninth rib.

The lateral projection is key when working out at what levels the splanchnic branches arise as well as their cranio-caudal angulation for catheter placement. Therefore any planning for mesenteric angiography should be undertaken on a preceding CT.

4.20 PA chest radiograph

Please note the side marker!

(a) Left pericardial fat pad. This is of no clinical bearing but can sometimes be confused for a mediastinal mass because of its shape. The density of a fat pad is less than that produced by soft tissue mass lesions.
(b) Left main bronchus.
(c) Right first rib.
(d) Right costophrenic angle.
(e) Situs inversus. The radiograph has been presented the wrong way round but the side marker is present on the film.

Situs inversus implies the position of the heart is mirrored as is that of the abdominal viscera. Normal position is referred to as situs solitus.

If solely the position of the heart is altered, with the apex towards the right, then this is referred to as dextrocardia.

Kartagener's syndrome is a not infrequent association with situs inversus, affecting 20% of patients. It is a disease affecting mucociliary function and therefore patients often present with sinusitis and bronchiectasis.

Situs inversus also has bearing on patients presenting with trauma or abdominal pain and it needs to be considered, for instance, the spleen will be on the right and the appendix on the left.

Examination 5: Questions

Case 5.1

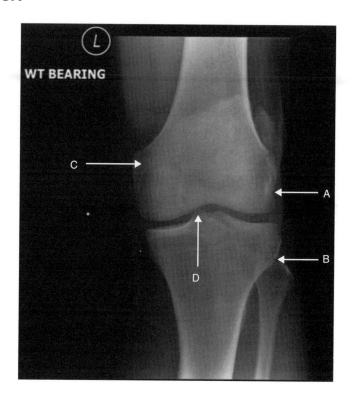

	QUESTION	WRITE YOUR ANSWER HERE
(a)	Name the structure that inserts at the point labelled A.	
(b)	Name the structure labelled B.	
(c)	Name the structure that attaches at the point labelled C.	
(d)	Name the structure labelled D.	
(e)	Which normal variant is present on this image?	

Case 5.2

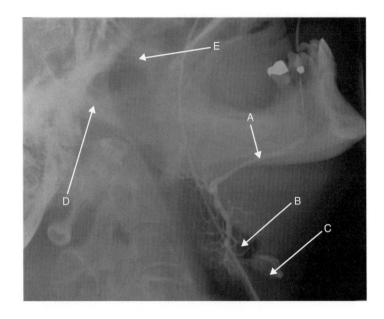

	QUESTION	WRITE YOUR ANSWER HERE
(a)	Name the structure labelled A.	
(b)	Name the structure labelled B.	
(c)	Name the structure labelled C.	
(d)	Name the structure labelled D.	
(e)	Name the structure labelled E.	

Case 5.3

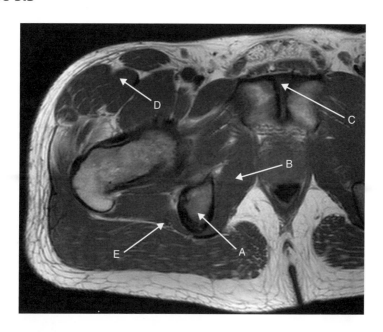

	QUESTION	WRITE YOUR ANSWER HERE
(a)	Name the structure labelled A.	
(b)	Name the structure labelled B.	
(c)	Name the structure labelled C.	
(d)	Name the structure labelled D.	
(e)	Name the structure labelled E.	

Case 5.4

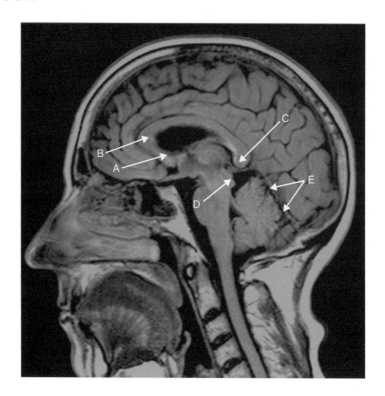

	QUESTION	WRITE YOUR ANSWER HERE
(a)	Name the structure labelled A.	
(b)	Name the structure labelled B.	
(c)	Name the structure labelled C.	
(d)	Name the structure labelled D.	
(e)	Name the structure labelled E.	

Case 5.5

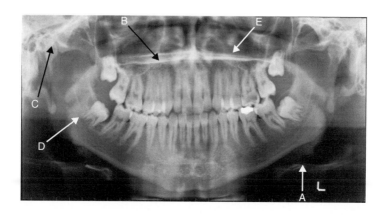

	QUESTION	WRITE YOUR ANSWER HERE
(a)	Name the structure labelled A.	
(b)	Name the structure labelled B.	
(c)	Name the structure labelled C.	
(d)	Name the structure labelled D.	
(e)	Name the structure labelled E.	

Case 5.6

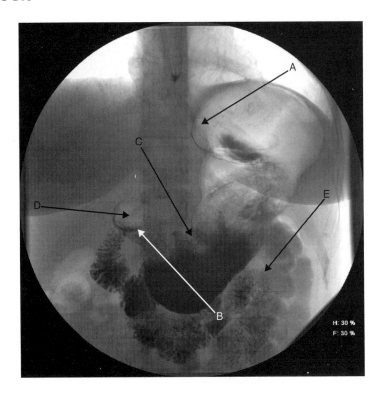

	QUESTION	WRITE YOUR ANSWER HERE
(a)	Name the structure labelled A.	
(b)	Name the structure labelled B.	
(c)	Name the structure labelled C.	
(d)	Name the structure labelled D.	
(e)	Name the structure labelled E.	

Case 5.7

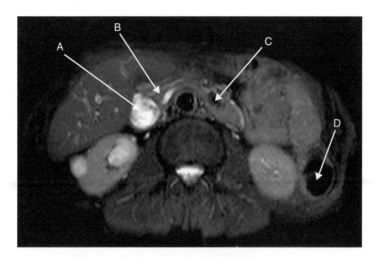

	QUESTION	WRITE YOUR ANSWER HERE
(a)	Name the structure labelled A.	
(b)	Name the structure labelled B.	
(c)	Name the structure labelled C.	
(d)	Name the structure labelled D.	
(e)	Name the normal variant present on this image?	

Case 5.8

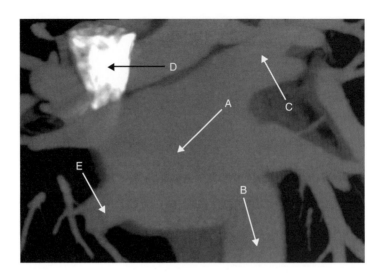

	QUESTION	WRITE YOUR ANSWER HERE
(a)	Name the structure labelled A.	
(b)	Name the structure labelled B.	
(c)	Name the structure labelled C.	
(d)	Name the structure labelled D.	
(e)	Name the structure labelled E.	

Case 5.9

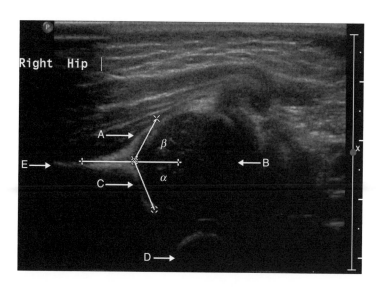

	QUESTION	WRITE YOUR ANSWER HERE
(a)	Name the structure labelled A.	
(b)	Name the structure labelled B.	
(c)	Name the structure labelled C.	
(d)	Name the structure labelled D.	
(e)	Name the structure labelled E.	

Case 5.10

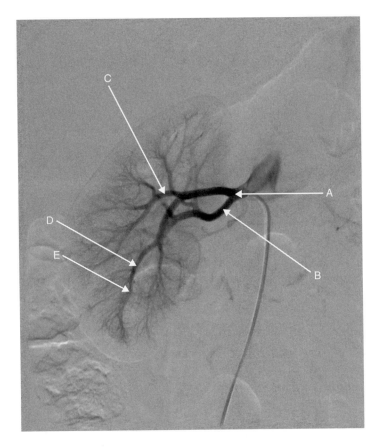

	QUESTION	WRITE YOUR ANSWER HERE
(a)	Name the structure labelled A.	
(b)	Name the structure labelled B.	
(c)	Name the structure labelled C.	
(d)	Name the structure labelled D.	
(e)	Name the structure labelled E.	

Case 5.11

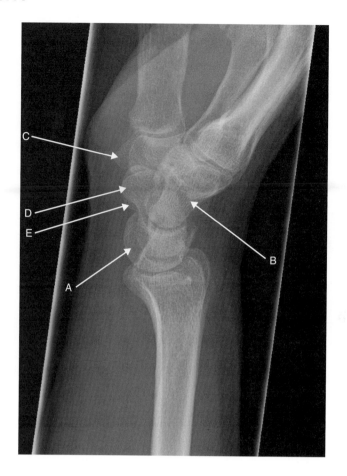

	QUESTION	WRITE YOUR ANSWER HERE
(a)	Name the structure labelled A.	
(b)	Name the structure labelled B.	
(c)	Name the structure labelled C.	
(d)	Name the structure labelled D.	
(e)	Name the structure labelled E.	

Case 5.12

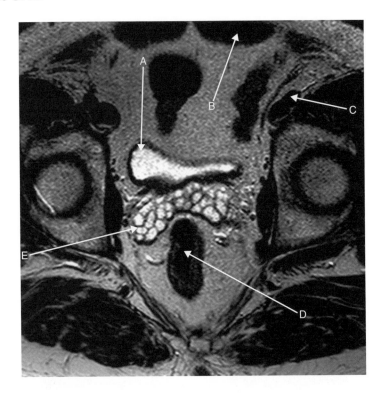

	QUESTION	WRITE YOUR ANSWER HERE
(a)	Name the structure labelled A.	
(b)	Name the structure labelled B.	
(c)	Name the structure labelled C.	
(d)	Name the structure labelled D.	
(e)	Name the structure labelled E.	

Case 5.13

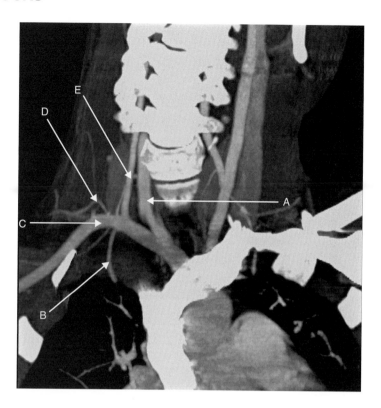

	QUESTION	WRITE YOUR ANSWER HERE
(a)	Name the structure labelled A.	
(b)	Name the structure labelled B.	
(c)	Name the structure labelled C.	
(d)	Name the structure labelled D.	
(e)	Name the structure labelled E.	

Case 5.14

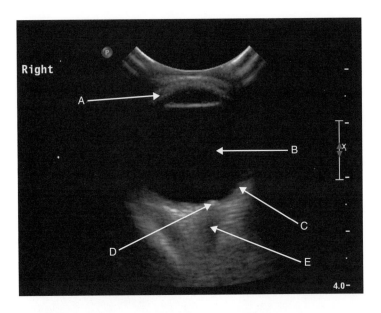

	QUESTION	WRITE YOUR ANSWER HERE
(a)	Name the structure labelled A.	
(b)	Name the structure labelled B.	
(c)	Name the structure labelled C.	
(d)	Name the structure labelled D.	
(e)	Name the structure labelled E.	

Case 5.15

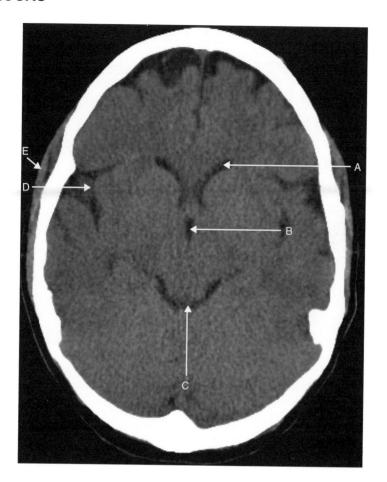

	QUESTION	WRITE YOUR ANSWER HERE
(a)	Name the structure labelled A.	
(b)	Name the structure labelled B.	
(c)	Name the structure labelled C.	
(d)	Name the structure labelled D.	
(e)	Name the structure labelled E.	

Case 5.16

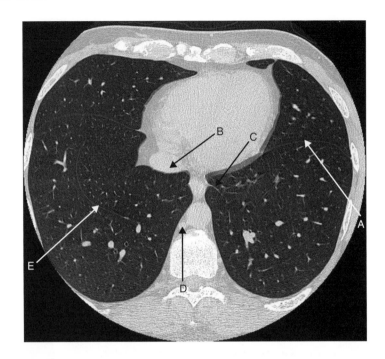

	QUESTION	WRITE YOUR ANSWER HERE
(a)	Name the structure labelled A.	
(b)	Name the structure labelled B.	
(c)	Name the structure labelled C.	
(d)	Name the structure labelled D.	
(e)	Name the structure labelled E.	

Case 5.17

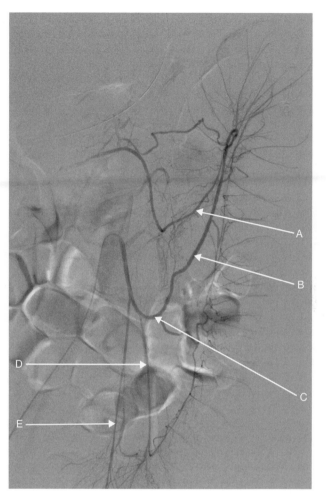

	QUESTION	WRITE YOUR ANSWER HERE
(a)	Name the structure labelled A.	
(b)	Name the structure labelled B.	
(c)	Name the structure labelled C.	
(d)	Name the structure labelled D.	
(e)	Name the structure labelled E.	

Case 5.18

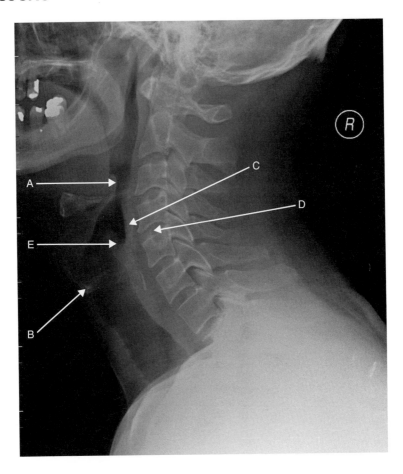

	QUESTION	WRITE YOUR ANSWER HERE
(a)	Name the structure labelled A.	
(b)	Name the structure labelled B.	
(c)	Name the structure labelled C.	
(d)	Name the structure labelled D.	
(e)	Name the structure labelled E.	

Case 5.19

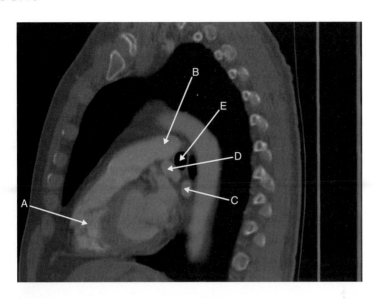

	QUESTION	WRITE YOUR ANSWER HERE
(a)	Name the structure labelled A.	
(b)	Name the structure labelled B.	
(c)	Name the structure labelled C.	
(d)	Name the structure labelled D.	
(e)	Name the structure labelled E.	

Case 5.20

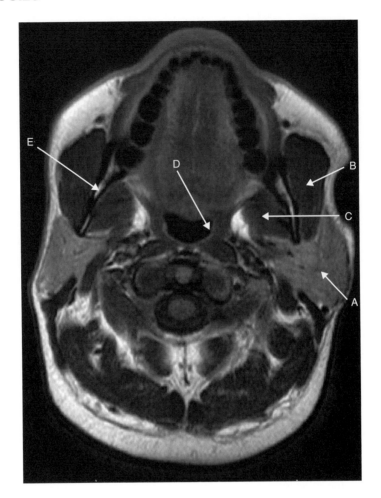

	QUESTION	WRITE YOUR ANSWER HERE
(a)	Name the structure labelled A.	
(b)	Name the structure labelled B.	
(c)	Name the structure labelled C.	
(d)	Name the structure labeled D.	
(e)	Name the structure labeled E.	

Examination 5: Answers

5.1 AP radiograph left knee

(a) Popliteus tendon. This point represents the popliteal groove or sulcus within which the popliteus tendon inserts. The popliteus tendon is an important structure that contributes to stability of the postero-lateral corner of the knee.

(b) Styloid process of the fibular head. Biceps femoris, a powerful hamstring muscle, attaches here along with the fibular collateral ligament and the arcuate ligament complex. The fibular styloid process can be avulsed during high energy trauma to the postero-lateral corner of the knee producing an 'arcuate sign' on radiographs.

(c) Medial collateral ligament (MCL). The MCL is an important medial stabilizer of the knee, resisting valgus stress. A bony avulsion of the proximal MCL attachment may produce a non-united fragment called a Pellegrini–Stieda lesion, visible on AP radiographs.

(d) Medial tibial spine. The medial tibial spine bears the attachment of the medial meniscal roots along with the footprint of the antero-medial bundle of the anterior cruciate ligament.

(e) Bipartite patella. A bipartite patella is an unfused secondary ossification centre on the supero-lateral corner of the patella. These must not be mistaken for acute fractures, but may become symptomatic if the synchondrosis between the two bone fragments is disrupted following direct trauma.

5.2 Sialogram

(a) Main submandibular duct. This is also known as Wharton's duct, and conveys mixed mucinous and serous secretions, which are more prone to form opaque calculi.

(b) Intraglandular duct. On ultrasound scan examination, intraglandular ducts are visualized as small linear hypoechoic stripes.

(c) Hyoid bone. This does not articulate with any other bone, and is held in position by the thyroid ligaments. It is highly mobile, with mobility provided by a number of muscles and ligaments. It develops from the second and third pharyngeal arches.

(d) Condylar process of the mandible. The lateral extremity of the condyle is a small tubercle for the attachment of the temporomandibular ligament.

(e) Coronoid process of the mandible. This is a thin triangular eminence, whose lateral surface affords insertion to the temporalis and masseter muscles.

5.3 Axial T1-weighted MR right hip

(a) Right ischial tuberosity. The tendons of semi-membranosus, semi-tendinosus and biceps femoris originate from the ischial tuberosity. Traumatic avulsion of the hamstring origin may be seen in sprinting and kicking sports.

(b) Right obturator internus muscle. The obturator internus arises from the internal surface of the obturator ring and inserts on the medial surface of the greater trochanter. Its action is to laterally rotate the hip and abduct the thigh when the hip is in flexion. Tumours of the rectum and ischio-rectal fossa may invade this muscle.

(c) Symphysis pubis. This is a type II fibrocartilaginous joint between the pubic bones. It resists pelvis rotation and anterior compression and thus may become disrupted during pelvic trauma following these mechanisms, resulting in symphyseal diastasis or malalignment. If missed this leads to pelvic instability and symphyseal pain.

(d) Right rectus femoris. This is an important muscle that contributes to hip flexion and knee extension. It arises from the anterior inferior iliac spine (AIIS) and in the immature skeleton the AIIS apophysis may become avulsed during kicking sports such as football. Injury of this muscle–tendon unit in adulthood usually presents with tearing at the musculo-tendinous junction.

(e) Right sciatic nerve. This is the largest nerve in the body made up of the L4, L5, S1 and S2 roots. In the region shown in the image the sciatic nerve may undergo entrapment by the piriformis muscle, which runs superficial to the nerve. This is known as 'piriformis syndrome' and may mimic other causes of sciatic neuropathy such as L5/S1 disc herniation, hence the alternative name of 'pseudosciatica'.

5.4 Sagittal MR brain (FLAIR sequence)

(a) Rostrum of the corpus callosum. This is the first part of the corpus callosum which extends from the anterior commissure.

(b) Genu of the corpus callosum. This is the most anterior part of the corpus callosum where it bends sharply backwards. Fibres extending from the genu into the frontal cortex are called forceps minor.

(c) Splenium of the corpus callosum. This is the thickened posterior end of the corpus callosum. Fibres extending posteriorly from the splenium into the occipital lobes are called forceps major.

(d) Quadrigeminal plate. This is also known as the tectum, and forms part of the midbrain lying posterior to the cerebral aqueduct (of Sylvius).

(e) Tentorium cerebelli. This is an extension of dura mater, separating the cerebellum from the inferior portion of the occipital lobes. The upper surface, in the midline, attaches to the posterior surface of the falx cerebri and the straight sinus runs in this location.

5.5 OPG (orthopantomogram)

(a) Hyoid bone. This lies at the level of C3 and consists of a body and superior and inferior cornu.

(b) Hard palate. Three foramina open onto the oral surface of the hard palate – the incisive fossa and the greater and lesser palatine foramina.

(c) Right mandibular condyle. The anterior projection of the ramus is called the coronoid process.

(d) Right inferior alveolar canal. This transmits the inferior alveolar vessels and nerve which are branches of the maxillary vessels and nerves. The proximal opening is the mandibular foramen on the inner surface of the ramus. Distally the canal opens at the mental foramen on the external surface of the body between the two premolars.

(e) Left maxillary sinus. The maxillary sinus opens via the ostium into the infundibulum.

OPGs are taken by a moving x-ray source and film. The trajectory that the x-ray source describes is that of a hemicircle behind the patient's head while the moving film mechanism remains diametrically opposite, anterior to the patient's face.

The primary use of the OPG is to assess dentition although mandibular pathology can also be diagnosed. Its advantage is that it allows broad coverage of the teeth and facial bones in a short acquisition time.

5.6 Barium meal

(a) Gastric cardia. The gastric cardia is well seen on double contrast barium studies. A variety of appearances may be seen, such as a filling defect, radiating folds of the cardiac rosette and hooded fold.

(b) Pylorus. This is usually located at the L1 level to the right of the midline.

(c) Angular incisura. This demarcation along the lesser curve of the stomach separates the body from the pylorus.

(d) Superior or first part of the duodenum. Lies antero-lateral to the L1 vertebra. The first part (2 cm in length) has a mesentery and is mobile. This is known as the duodenal cap.

(e) Duodeno-jejunal (DJ) flexure junction. This is situated on the left side approximately at the level of L2 vertebra, 2–3 cm left of the midline.

5.7 Axial T2-weighted abdominal MR (fat-suppressed sequence)

(a) Second part of duodenum (or D2). The pancreatic head has a constant relationship with the duodenum. The right lateral border is nestled in the duodenal sweep.

(b) Dorsal pancreatic duct (of Santorini).

(c) Superior mesenteric artery (SMA). Flow void is seen in the SMA as it courses over the uncinate process of the pancreas. It arises 1–2 cm below the coeliac axis typically at the level of L1.

(d) Descending colon.

(e) Pancreatic divisum. This is the most common variant of pancreatic ductal fusion and drainage anomalies. It is caused by failure of fusion of the dorsal and ventral buds. The short ventral duct of Wirsung drains the head and uncinate process, with the long dorsal pancreatic duct of Santorini draining the body and tail. It is typically seen in up to 6% of the population and up to 25% of patients with idiopathic pancreatitis, though it is not proven to be a causative mechanism.

Incidentally, there are two high signal cysts seen in the right kidney.

5.8 Cardiac CT

(a) Left atrium.
(b) Descending thoracic aorta.
(c) Left superior pulmonary vein.
(d) Superior vena cava.
(e) Right inferior pulmonary vein.

Normal pulmonary venous anatomy consists of a superior and inferior pulmonary veins on each side, draining into the left atrium. It is important to remember these carry oxygenated blood.

In addition to the normal pulmonary veins on the right, there may also be one or two middle pulmonary veins and/or an upper pulmonary vein draining into the superior surface of the left atrium. On the left, the superior and inferior pulmonary veins may join to form a common trunk, either short or long. All these variant veins drain directly into the left atrium.

At the root of the lung, the superior pulmonary vein lies anterior and inferior to the pulmonary artery while the inferior pulmonary vein lies in the inferior part of the lung hilum.

5.9 Paediatric right hip ultrasound

(a) Labrum.
(b) Femoral head.
(c) Acetabulum.
(d) Pubis.
(e) Ileum.

The beta (β) angle of the hip is the angle of the fibrocartilage to the ilium and the alpha (α) angle is the angle of depth of the bony acetabulum. The normal angles are:

α >60 degrees
β <77 degrees.

These angles are important to define the presence and severity of congenital hip dysplasia. The Graf classification indicates the degree of congenital hip dysplasia.

5.10 Right renal angiogram

(a) Right renal artery. The renal arteries arise from the aorta approximately at the upper margin of L2. Sixty-five per cent of kidneys are supplied by a solitary vessel; 35% have an aberrant vascular supply. The right renal artery is usually longer and passes behind the inferior vena cava.

The most sensitive and specific non-invasive screening test for renal vessel disease is MRA (98% and 100% respectively) followed by CT (92% and 83%) and duplex ultrasound (89% and 97%).

(b) Posterior division of the renal artery.
(c) Segmental artery.
(d) Interlobar artery. These arteries lie between the lobes (or pyramids) of the kidney.
(e) Arcuate artery. These arteries do not anastamose to form arcades, but run along the base of the pyramids.

The branching pattern from the aorta is therefore:
Main renal artery – anterior and posterior division – segmental arteries – interlobar arteries – arcuate arteries.

Between the anterior and posterior divisions of the renal artery is the plane of Brodel, which is at the postero-lateral approach to the kidney. It is relatively avascular and is the plane targeted for when performing percutaneous nephrostomy.

5.11 Lateral wrist radiograph

(a) Lunate.
(b) Capitate.
(c) Trapezoid.
(d) Scaphoid.
(e) Pisiform.

5.12 Axial T2-weighted MR male pelvis

(a) Urinary bladder. Fluid is seen as high signal on T2-weighted and low signal on T1-weighted images, unless it is haemorrhagic or proteinaceous when it will be high on T1-weighted images. The wall of the urinary bladder should be clearly defined and <5 mm in thickness when adequately distended.

(b) Left rectus abdominis muscle.

(c) Left femoral artery.

(d) Rectum.

(e) Right seminal vesicles. Seminal vesicles are seen as high signal on T2-weighted and low signal on T1-weighted images. It is essential to evaluate seminal vesicles when staging prostatic carcinoma, as disease involvement changes the staging and usually renders the patient inoperable. Tumour involvement will change the high T2 signal to low signal. When evaluating the MRI, ensure no haemorrhage is present in the seminal vesicles (from transrectal prostate biopsy) as this can lead to interpretation errors.

Seminal vesicles are paired sacculated diverticula that lie transversely posterior to the prostate and store seminal fluid. They narrow inferiorly to fuse with the vas deferens and become the ejaculatory ducts.

5.13 Oblique coronal maximum intensity projection (MIP) aortic arch vessels

(a) Right common carotid artery. This bifurcates at C4 level. It lies in the carotid sheath medial to the jugular vein with the vagus nerve interposed in between and posterior to them.

Neither the common carotid or internal carotid arteries have any other branches. The external carotid artery gives off seven branches.

Diseases of the carotid arteries are investigated using primarily Duplex ultrasound or MRA, or usually both if there is indeterminate pathology.

(b) Right internal thoracic (or mammary) artery.

(c) Right subclavian artery. The right subclavian and carotid arteries arise from the innominate (or brachiocephalic) artery. There is no equivalent on the contralateral side where the two vessels have a separate origin from the aortic arch.

The subclavian artery lies in a groove in the superior surface of the first rib behind the subclavian vein, the two being separated by the scalene muscle, which divides the artery, into three parts. At the outer border of the first rib it becomes the axillary artery which in turn becomes the brachial artery at the lower border of teres major.

(d) Right thyrocervical trunk.

(e) Right vertebral artery. This vessel acts as a bypass conduit in subclavian steal syndrome where the ostium of the subclavian artery is blocked. The upper limb is then perfused via retrograde blood flow down the vertebral artery from the cerebral circulation.

5.14 Ultrasound orbit

(a) Cornea. The most superficial structure apparent is the eyelid. The next interface marks the thin layer of fluid over and bathing the cornea.

(b) Vitreous humour. This is contained in the posterior chamber of the eye. Between the two chambers lie the iris, lens, suspensory ligaments and ciliary muscles.

(c) Retina.

(d) Optic disc. The layers of the globe internal to external are the retina, the choroid and the sclera.

(e) Optic nerve. The optic nerve is normally less than 5mm in diameter, if it is greater than this then raised intracranial pressure or an expansive lesion of the optic nerve may be present.

Ultrasound of the eye is performed with the lid closed using an ultrasound gel cushion to avoid unnecessary pressure on the globe. The high spatial resolution of ultrasound makes it particularly good for assessing the globe.

5.15 Axial unenhanced CT brain

(a) Anterior horn of the left lateral ventricle. The lateral ventricles are C-shaped cavities which sit below the corpus callosum, consisting of a body, anterior and temporal horns. They drain into the third ventricle via the interventricular foramina of Monro (one on each side).

(b) Third ventricle. The cerebrospinal fluid (CSF) drains from the third to fourth ventricle via the cerebral aqueduct (of Sylvius). The fourth ventricle empties into the central canal of the spinal cord or the subarachnoid space via the foramen of Magendie (centrally) and the two foramina of Lushka (laterally). CSF is absorbed from the subarachnoid space via the arachnoid villi which project out of the superior sagittal sinus.

(c) Quadrigeminal cistern. This is one of a series of cisterns which lie within the subarachnoid space, around the base of the brain and brainstem. Given the circle of Willis lies within this space, a subtle subarachnoid haemorrhage may only be apparent here, either as high attenuation within one of the cisternal spaces, effacing the Sylvian fissure or layered posteriorly in the lateral or fourth ventricles.

(d) Right Sylvian fissure.

(e) Right temporalis muscle.

5.16 Axial CT thorax (lung windows)

(a) Left oblique (major) fissure.

(b) Inferior vena cava.

(c) Left inferior pulmonary ligament or left pulmonary ligament. The pulmonary ligament is present bilaterally and comprises two pleural layers that extend downwards from the hilum of the lung between the inferior part of the mediastinal surface of the lung and the pericardium, joining the medial lower lobe to the mediastinum and diaphragm. It is situated inferior to the inferior pulmonary vein.

(d) Azygos vein.

(e) Right inferior accessory fissure. The right inferior accessory fissure is detected with high resolution CT (HRCT) in approximately 20% of patients. It is seen in 8% of PA chest radiographs and will only be detected if the x-ray beam is tangential to the fissure. It separates the medial basal segment from the rest of the right lower lobe. Note: the incidence of accessory fissures varies widely from study to study.

Consolidation in the medial basal segment of the right lower lobe may have a clear demarcation line at the site of this fissure.

Other accessory fissures are:

Azygos fissure – 1–4% of PA chest radiographs (depending on study)
Superior accessory fissure – 5% of PA chest radiographs
Left minor fissure – 2% of PA chest radiographs.

5.17 Inferior mesenteric angiogram

(a) Arc of Riolan. This vessel lies in the mesentery and provides a connection between the superior mesenteric artery (SMA) and inferior mesenteric artery (IMA) via the middle and left colic arteries at the splenic flexure. There is a more peripheral connection of the intestinal arcades which parallel the bowel wall; in the small bowel this is called the marginal artery of Dwight and in the colon it is called the marginal artery of Drummond.

(b) Ascending branch of the left colic artery.

(c) Left colic artery.

(d) Sigmoid arteries.

(e) Superior haemorrhoidal (rectal) artery. The superior haemorrhoidal artery is a continuation of the inferior mesenteric artery and branches from it communicate with the middle haemorrhoidal (rectal) artery, which arises from the internal iliac artery and is one of three potential collateral pathways that allow lower limb perfusion in aortic occlusion:

1. Aorta – SMA – IMA – superior haemorrhoidals – internal pudendal artery – internal iliac artery – external iliac artery.
2. Aorta – lumbar artery – ilio-lumbar – internal iliac – external iliac.
3. Aorta – posterior intercostal and lumbar arteries – deep circumflex iliac artery – external iliac artery.

5.18 Lateral C-spine radiograph

(a) Epiglottis. The epiglottis is a thin strip of cartilage attached inferiorly to the thyroid cartilage. During swallowing it covers the entrance of the larynx. It is attached on either side via pharyngeal folds to the lateral walls of the pharynx. Three anteriorly placed glosso-epiglottic folds attach to the base of the tongue and the spaces between the folds give rise to the valleculae.

(b) Anterior arch of cricoid cartilage. The cricoid cartilage has a ring structure anteriorly and a flat surface posteriorly. The cricothyroid membrane joins the cricoid and thyroid cartilages.

(c) Superior cornu of thyroid cartilage. The thyroid cartilage forms the antero-lateral laryngeal borders. There is a notch anteriorly at C4 level known as the superior thyroid notch. Posteriorly the laminae of the thyroid cartilage form horns – the superior cornu, which joins with the posterior hyoid bone via the triticeal cartilage in the lateral thyrohyoid ligament, and the inferior cornu, which articulates with the cricoid cartilage.

(d) Anterior tubercle of transverse process of C5.

(e) Thyroid cartilage.

5.19 Sagittal thorax CT

(a) Right ventricle.
(b) Pulmonary trunk.
(c) Left inferior pulmonary vein.
(d) Left superior pulmonary vein.
(e) Left main bronchus. The left main bronchus has a more horizontal course than the right main bronchus. Consequently the left main bronchus is ovoid on lateral chest radiographs and sagittal CT images, unlike the right main bronchus, which is tubular and more 'vertical'.

5.20 Axial T1-weighted MR of the neck

(a) Left parotid gland. This is the largest salivary gland and is divided into deep and superficial lobes which are connected around the posterior surface of the mandible by the isthmus. Its duct (Stensen's duct) opens into the buccal cavity opposite the upper second molar tooth.

(b) Left masseter muscle. This muscle lies in the masseteric space with the pterygoid muscles. It has deep and superficial components and is innervated by a branch of the mandibular nerve (trigeminal nerve III). The space is an important tissue compartment in the face and can be the site of abscess formation. It is often difficult to diagnose pathology here.

(c) Left pterygoid muscles. The medial pterygoid muscle extends from the pterygoid plates medially to the inner surface of the mandibular condyle laterally. The medial pterygoid inserts with the masseter by a common tendinous sling onto the medial surface of the ramus and angle of the mandible. It thus contributes to elevation of the jaw. The lateral pterygoid muscle arises from the greater wing of the sphenoid bone, and the lateral surface of the lateral pterygoid plate. It inserts onto the mandibular condyle with its superior head attaching onto the articular disc and fibrous capsule of the temporomandibular joint. It acts by lowering the mandible and so opens the jaw. Unilateral action of a lateral pterygoid produces contralateral excursion and so contributes to chewing.

(d) Left lateral wall of the pharynx. Lateral to this lies fat in the left parapharyngeal space which is seen as high signal on this T1-weighted image.

(e) Right ramus of the mandible. The fatty marrow appears bright and the cortex dark on this T1-weighted image.

Examination 6: Questions

Case 6.1

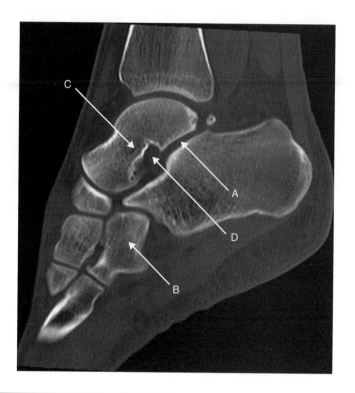

	QUESTION	WRITE YOUR ANSWER HERE
(a)	Name the joint labelled A.	
(b)	Name the structure labelled B.	
(c)	Name the structure labelled C.	
(d)	Name the structure labelled D.	
(e)	Which normal variant is present on this image?	

Case 6.2

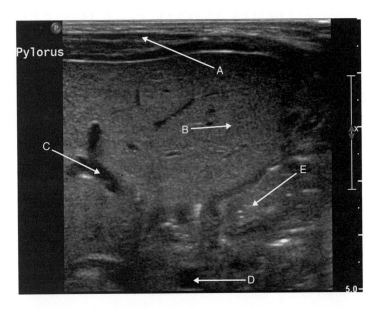

	QUESTION	WRITE YOUR ANSWER HERE
(a)	Name the structure labelled A.	
(b)	Name the structure labelled B.	
(c)	Name the structure labelled C.	
(d)	Name the structure labelled D.	
(e)	Name the structure labelled E.	

Case 6.3

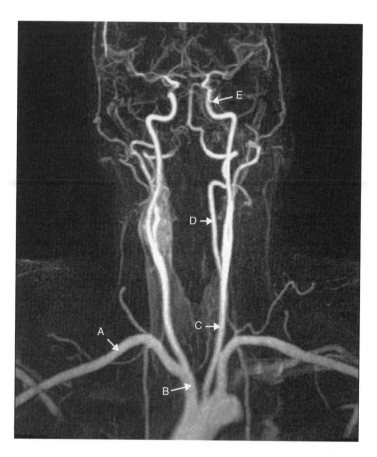

	QUESTION	WRITE YOUR ANSWER HERE
(a)	Name the structure labelled A.	
(b)	Name the structure labelled B.	
(c)	Name the structure labelled C.	
(d)	Name the structure labelled D.	
(e)	Name the structure labelled E.	

Case 6.4

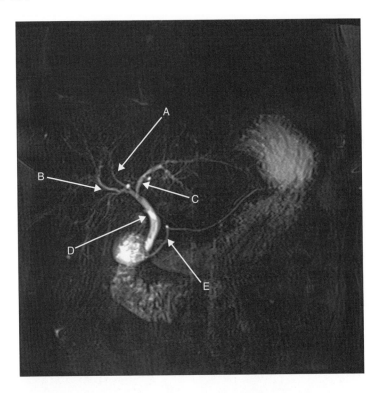

	QUESTION	WRITE YOUR ANSWER HERE
(a)	Name the structure labelled A.	
(b)	Name the structure labelled B.	
(c)	Name the structure labelled C.	
(d)	Name the structure labelled D.	
(e)	Name the structure labelled E.	

Case 6.5

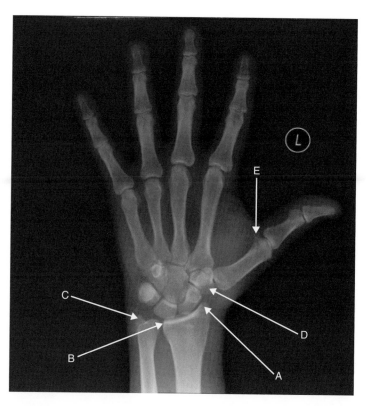

	QUESTION	WRITE YOUR ANSWER HERE
(a)	Name the structure labelled A.	
(b)	Name the structure labelled B.	
(c)	Name the structure labelled C.	
(d)	Name the structure labelled D.	
(e)	Name the structure in which the sesamoid bone labelled E lies.	

Case 6.6

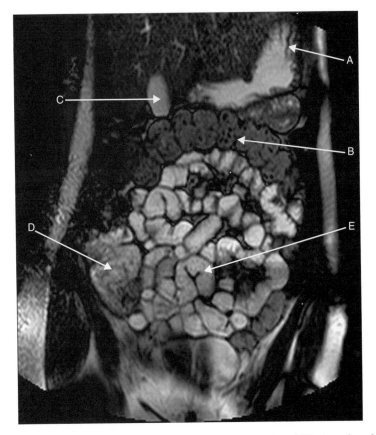

Image courtesy of Priya Healey, Consultant Radiologist, Royal Liverpool and Broadgreen University Hospital, Liverpool, UK.

	QUESTION	WRITE YOUR ANSWER HERE
(a)	Name the structure labelled A.	
(b)	Name the structure labelled B.	
(c)	Name the structure labelled C.	
(d)	Name the structure labelled D.	
(e)	Name the structure labelled E.	

Case 6.7

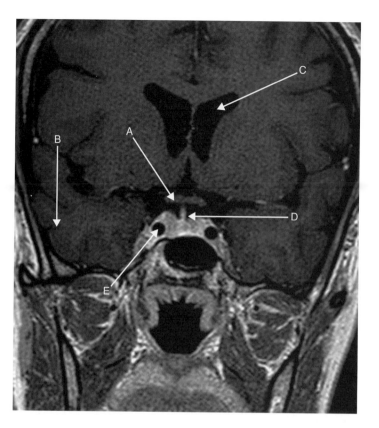

	QUESTION	WRITE YOUR ANSWER HERE
(a)	Name the structure labelled A.	
(b)	Name the structure labelled B.	
(c)	Name the structure labelled C.	
(d)	Name the structure labelled D.	
(e)	Name the structure labelled E.	

Case 6.8

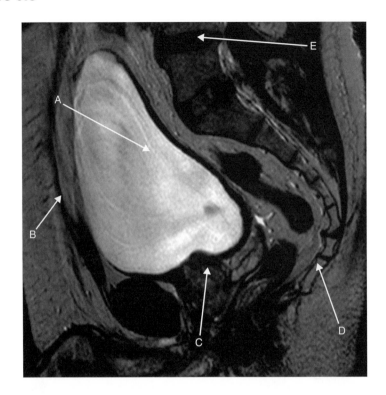

	QUESTION	WRITE YOUR ANSWER HERE
(a)	Name the structure labelled A.	
(b)	Name the structure labelled B.	
(c)	Name the structure labelled C.	
(d)	Name the structure labelled D.	
(e)	Name the structure labelled E.	

Case 6.9

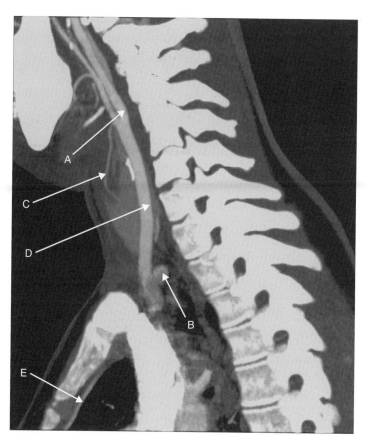

	QUESTION	WRITE YOUR ANSWER HERE
(a)	Name the structure labelled A.	
(b)	Name the structure labelled B.	
(c)	Name the structure labelled C.	
(d)	Name the structure labelled D.	
(e)	Name the structure labelled E.	

Case 6.10

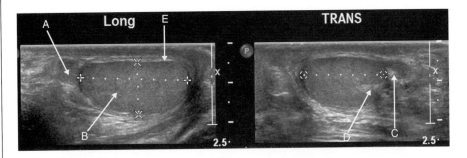

	QUESTION	WRITE YOUR ANSWER HERE
(a)	Name the structure labelled A.	
(b)	Name the structure labelled B.	
(c)	Name the structure labelled C.	
(d)	Name the structure labelled D.	
(e)	Name the structure labelled E.	

Case 6.11

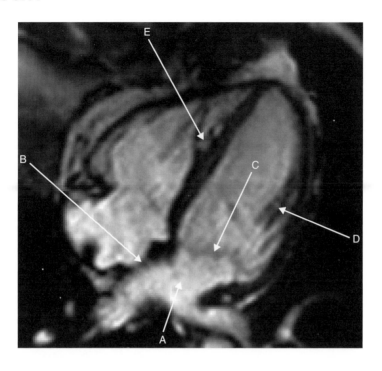

	QUESTION	WRITE YOUR ANSWER HERE
(a)	Name the structure labelled A.	
(b)	Name the structure labelled B.	
(c)	Name the structure labelled C.	
(d)	Name the structure labelled D.	
(e)	Name the structure labelled E.	

Case 6.12

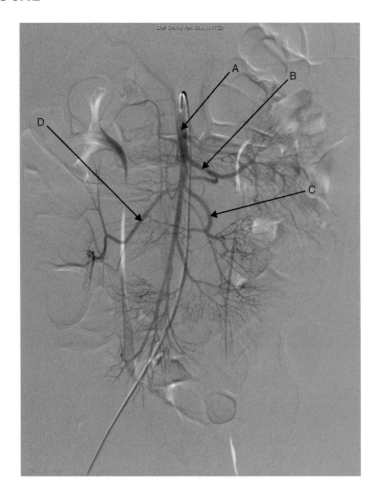

	QUESTION	WRITE YOUR ANSWER HERE
(a)	Name the structure labelled A.	
(b)	Name the structure labelled B.	
(c)	Name the structure labelled C.	
(d)	Name the structure labelled D.	
(e)	Which normal variant is present on this image?	

Case 6.13

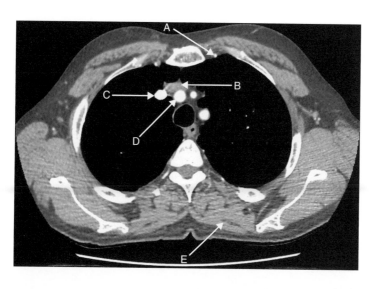

	QUESTION	WRITE YOUR ANSWER HERE
(a)	Name the structure labelled A.	
(b)	Name the structure labelled B.	
(c)	Name the structure labelled C.	
(d)	Name the structure labelled D.	
(e)	Name the structure labelled E.	

Case 6.14

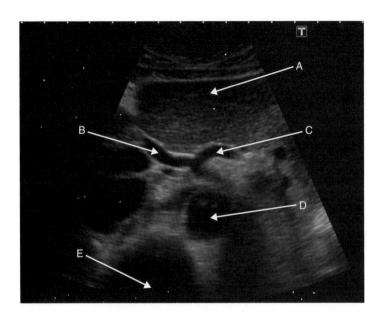

	QUESTION	WRITE YOUR ANSWER HERE
(a)	Name the structure labelled A.	
(b)	Name the structure labelled B.	
(c)	Name the structure labelled C.	
(d)	Name the structure labelled D.	
(e)	Name the structure labelled E.	

Case 6.15

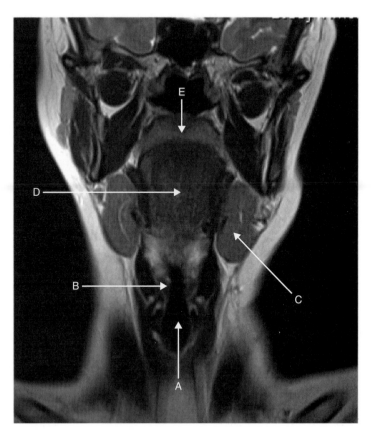

	QUESTION	WRITE YOUR ANSWER HERE
(a)	Name the structure labelled A.	
(b)	Name the structure labelled B.	
(c)	Name the structure labelled C.	
(d)	Name the structure labelled D.	
(e)	Name the structure labelled E.	

Case 6.16

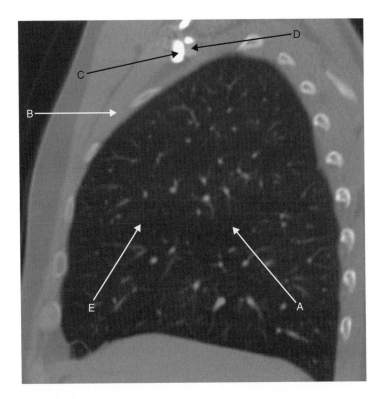

	QUESTION	WRITE YOUR ANSWER HERE
(a)	Name the structure labelled A.	
(b)	Name the structure labelled B.	
(c)	Name the structure labelled C.	
(d)	Name the structure labelled D.	
(e)	Name the structure labelled E.	

Case 6.17

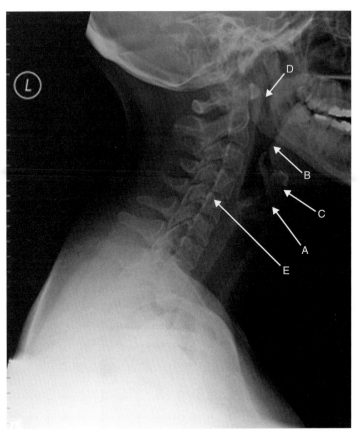

	QUESTION	WRITE YOUR ANSWER HERE
(a)	Name the structure labelled A.	
(b)	Name the structure labelled B.	
(c)	Name the structure labelled C.	
(d)	Name the structure labelled D.	
(e)	Name the structure labelled E.	

Case 6.18

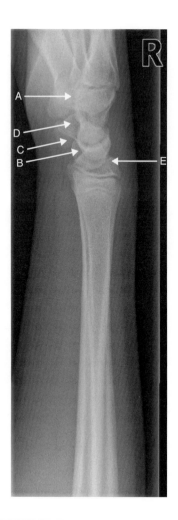

	QUESTION	WRITE YOUR ANSWER HERE
(a)	Name the structure labelled A.	
(b)	Name the structure labelled B.	
(c)	Name the structure labelled C.	
(d)	Name the structure labelled D.	
(e)	Name the structure labelled E.	

Case 6.19

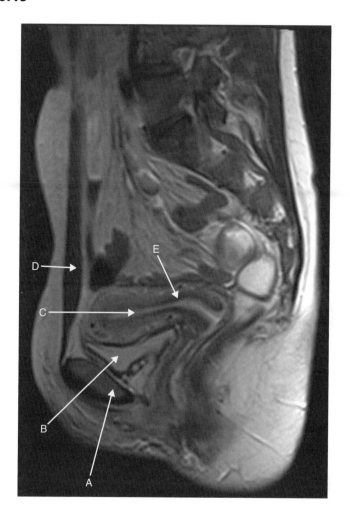

	QUESTION	WRITE YOUR ANSWER HERE
(a)	Name the structure labelled A.	
(b)	Name the structure labelled B.	
(c)	Name the structure labelled C.	
(d)	Name the structure labelled D.	
(e)	Name the structure labelled E.	

Case 6.20

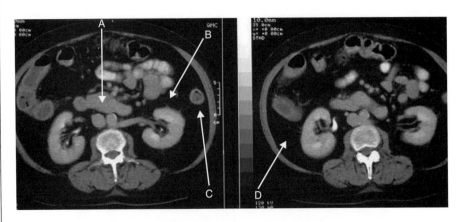

	QUESTION	WRITE YOUR ANSWER HERE
(a)	Name the structure labelled A.	
(b)	Name the structure labelled B.	
(c)	Name the structure labelled C.	
(d)	Name the structure labelled D.	
(e)	Which normal variant is present on this image?	

Examination 6: Answers

6.1 Sagittal CT ankle

(a) Posterior sub-talar joint (PSTJ). The PSTJ is a synovial joint formed by the articulation of the posterior articular facets of the talus and calcaneum. Intra-articular extension into the PSTJ is often seen in comminuted calcaneal compression fractures and represents an important factor in the surgical classification of these injuries.

(b) Cuboid. The cuboid possesses a proximal articular surface that only articulates with the calcaneum. Distally the cuboid articulates with the fourth and fifth metatarsals.

(c) Neck of the talus. The talar neck is an important review area when evaluating ankle radiographs and CT in the setting of trauma. Missed talar neck fractures can result in avascular necrosis of the talar dome due to its blood supply being derived from vessels that enter the talar head and travel proximally within the neck.

(d) The sinus tarsi. This is a fatty space beneath the talar neck and above the calcaneal body. The sinus tarsi also contains the cervical and interosseous ligaments along with traversing nerves and vessels. Inflammation and cyst formation in this space following trauma may produce a painful 'sinus-tarsi syndrome'.

(e) Os trigonum. This is present in 10% of individuals and when present, is bilateral in 50%. It may be present as a separate ossicle or be partly fused with the posterior talar process forming a synchrondrosis. The os trigonum may produce repetitive soft tissue impingment in the ankle due to repetitive plantar-flexion resulting in a painful 'os-trigonum syndrome'.

6.2 Transverse ultrasound through stomach pylorus and upper abdomen

(a) Rectus abdominus muscle.
(b) Left lobe of liver.
(c) Portal vein.
(d) Aorta.
(e) Pylorus.

In infants pyloric stenosis is diagnosed if the single wall thickness of the pylorus is greater than 6 mm and the pyloric length is greater than 17 mm.

The stomach will often be distended with feed despite projectile-type vomiting.

The pylorus is not seen open and there is no passage of stomach contents into the duodenum during scanning. Typically presentation is at about 6 weeks of life.

6.3 MRA carotids

(a) Right subclavian artery. This arises from the bifurcation of the brachiocephalic trunk behind the right sternoclavicular joint. An anomalous right subclavian artery occurs in 1% of the population.

(b) The brachiocephalic trunk. This bifurcates into the right common carotid and subclavian arteries and is the first major branch of the ascending aorta.

(c) Left common carotid artery. In 20% of the population this takes origin from the brachiocephalic trunk.

(d) Left vertebral artery. This travels through the transverse foramina of C6 to C1 where it passes medially to enter the foramen magnum.

(e) Left internal carotid artery. This begins at the level of C4 at the carotid bifurcation.

Imaging of the carotid arteries and other vessels with MR can largely be achieved without contrast. Either the signal from flowing blood entering an image plane can be measured (time of flight MRA) or the velocity differences in flowing blood can be measured (phase contrast MRA). However, these imaging techniques depend on laminar flow and therefore turbulent flow, as seen with stenoses, can result in signal loss and subsequent overestimation of stenoses and occlusion.

6.4 MRCP (magnetic resonance cholangiopancreatography)

MRCP of a post-cholecystectomy patient. Heavily T2-weighted maximum intensity projection (MIP) image of the biliary tree.

(a) Right anterior hepatic duct.
(b) Right posterior hepatic duct.
(c) Left hepatic duct.
(d) Common bile duct.
(e) Pancreatic duct.

Classical biliary tree anatomy occurs in about 58% of the population. The normal anatomy is the right hepatic duct and left hepatic duct draining the right and left lobes of the liver. The right hepatic duct branches into posterior duct draining segments VI and VII. The right posterior duct runs horizontally and posterior to the anterior duct and fuses to form the right hepatic duct. The anterior duct drains segments V and VIII. The left duct drains II–IV.

The commonest variant, in 15.6% of the population, is the right posterior duct draining into the left hepatic duct. The right anterior and posterior ducts fuse with the left to form a trifurcation in some people.

6.5 Dorso-palmar (DP) radiograph left hand

(a) Radial styloid process. This forms the dorsal and radial margins of the radio-carpal joint and may become fractured during forced radial and dorsal deviation of the wrist due to impaction by the scaphoid. This fracture was traditionally termed the 'chauffeur's fracture' due to the mechanism of injury sustained by turning a stiff crankshaft on old cars.

(b) Distal radio-ulnar joint (DRUJ). The DRUJ is a synovial joint formed by the sigmoid notch of the radius and the convex articular surface of the ulna. It is important as it facilitates wrist supination and pronation whilst the elbow is fixed. The distal margin of the joint is covered by the triangular fibrocartilage (TFC) and its supporting ligaments, thus TFC injury can lead to DRUJ instability.

(c) Ulnar styloid. The ulnar styloid projects distally from the dorsal aspect of the distal ulnar. It bears attachment of many important structures including the support-ing ligaments of the TFC and the sheath of the extensor carpi ulnaris tendon. It is commonly avulsed during wrist trauma by traction of these structures, which frequently results in fracture non-union.

(d) Trapezium. This forms a synovial saddle joint with the base of the metacarpal of the thumb. This joint is a common site for primary osteoarthritis due to its frequent use.

(e) Flexor pollicis longus (FPL). The paired FPL sesamoids are present in nearly all individuals and lie either side of the FPL tendon beneath the metacarpo-phalangeal (MCP) joint of the thumb. They are analogous to the paired flexor halluces longus (FHL) sesamoid bones found beneath the metatarso-phalangeal (MTP) joint of the hallux.

6.6 Coronal T2-weighted MR enteroclysis image

(a) Rugal folds of the stomach. When contracted the gastric mucosa is thrown into longitudinal ridges. They are most marked in the pyloric region and along the lesser curve.

(b) Transverse colon. Contains solid faecal matter and therefore on this T2-weighted fast field echo image appears of low signal mixed with air.

(c) Gallbladder. The bile shows as high signal on this T2-weighted image.

(d) Caecum. It appears high signal as there is still a certain amount of fluid within the faeces at this stage.

(e) Ileum. Note the wall is smooth and shows no obvious thickening or change in the surrounding tissue.

6.7 Coronal MRI pituitary

(a) Optic chiasm.

(b) Right middle temporal gyrus.

(c) Left lateral ventricle.

(d) Pituitary stalk.

(e) Right internal carotid artery in cavernous sinus. The cavernous sinus is a large thin-walled vein bordered by the temporal and sphenoid bones and lying lateral to the sella turcica. In addition to the internal carotid artery, the III, IV, V and VI cranial nerves also lie within the sinus.

Coronal MRI is useful for assessing the pituitary gland. When learning, a lot of radiologists think the sagittal sequence is more useful, but in practice the coronal sequence enables complete assessment of the pituitary when pre- and post-contrast T1-weighted sequences are obtained. The superior surface of the pituitary is concave or horizontal upwards. Any convexity upwards suggests a space-occupying lesion.

The pituitary stalk should lie in a central position and the pituitary gland should enhance uniformly. An area of pituitary that does not enhance may be caused by a pituitary microadenoma.

6.8 Sagittal T2-weighted MR pelvis (male)

(a) Urinary bladder.

(b) Rectus abdominis muscle.

(c) Prostate.

(d) Coccyx.

(e) L4/L5 intervertebral disc.

Thin sections are taken in all three planes when evaluating the prostate in order to ascertain if there is any extra-capsular disease.

MRI bladder includes dynamic, contrast-enhanced images as bladder tumours are hypervascular and show early enhancement. This ensures that correct staging can be performed. Sequences performed also include images of the upper tracts to ascertain if there is any hydronephrosis, hydroureter or ureteric tumour. CTU will often be performed in conjunction with MRI as transitional cell tumours can occur separately, both in the bladder and the upper tracts.

It is important to look at the entire image, even though it may be centred on a specific organ. Although T1-weighted images are optimum for evaluating bone marrow, look at the vertebral alignment on any sagittal images and for any intervertebral disc disease.

6.9 CT right carotid oblique MIP (maximum intensity projection) image

(a) Right internal carotid artery.
(b) Right internal thoracic artery.
(c) Right superior thyroid artery.
(d) Right common carotid artery (CCA).
(e) Right subclavian artery (SCA). It is difficult to ascertain this is the right side on this image. However, the anatomical relationship of the right SCA with the common carotid artery (CCA) is the clue.

6.10 Transverse and longitudinal ultrasound testis

(a) Epididymal head.
(b) Testis.
(c) Epididymal tail.
(d) Mediastinum testis.
(e) Tunica albuginea.

6.11 Cardiac MR

This image is a single frame from a 4-chamber cardiac MR white blood cine (steady state free precession) examination.

(a) Left atrium.
(b) Inter-atrial septum.
(c) Mitral valve.
(d) Papillary muscle.
(e) Moderator band. The right ventricle (RV) is more heavily trabeculated than the left and also has a thick muscular band running across the distal RV cavity from the septum to the base of the anterior papillary muscle. This is called the moderator band and carries the right bundle branch of the atrio-ventricular (AV) conduction system to the anterior papillary muscle. The moderator band is only seen in the RV and its presence is used to identify the RV on fetal echocardiogram.

6.12 Superior mesenteric artery arteriogram

(a) Superior mesenteric artery (SMA). This artery arises from the aorta at the level of the L1 vertebra. The inferior mesenteric artery arises from the anterior or left antero-lateral aspect of the aorta at L3 vertebral level.
(b) Jejunal branch of the SMA. There are usually between four and six jejunal branches.
(c) Ileal branch of the SMA. There are usually between 9 and 13 ileal branches which arise after the ileocolic artery.
(d) Right colic artery.

(e) Replaced right hepatic artery. The right hepatic has an aberrant origin from the SMA rather than from the common hepatic artery. (It is faintly visible rising diagonally to the right from close to the catheter tip.)

6.13 Contrast-enhanced CT thorax

(a) Left internal thoracic (mammary) artery.
(b) Left brachiocephalic vein.
(c) Superior vena cava.
(d) Brachiocephalic (innominate) trunk (artery).
(e) Left trapezius muscle.

6.14 Transverse ultrasound through the epigastrium

(a) Left lobe of the liver.
(b) Common hepatic artery. In normal subjects this may be difficult to see on colour Doppler because of its small diameter and tortuous course.
(c) Splenic artery. This is the largest branch of the coeliac trunk that follows a tortuous course posterior to omental bursa along the superior border of the pancreas.
(d) Aorta.
(e) Vertebral body. Typically the coeliac axis arises at the T12/L1 level.

6.15 Coronal T1-weighted MR oropharynx

(a) Subglottis. This is the area immediately below the cords and is an important area for assessing tumour spread in laryngeal carcinoma.
(b) Right vocal cord. The vocal cords are identified by their muscle signal intensity.
(c) Left submandibular gland. The normal gland appears of intermediate signal intensity compared with muscle on both T1-weighted and T2-weighted images.
(d) Midline septum of the tongue. This is high signal on T1-weighted and T2-weighted images due to fat content.
   This is an important landmark when staging tongue tumours to assess spread across the midline.
(e) Soft palate. This marks the division between the naso- and oropharynx.

6.16 Sagittal CT thorax

(a) Right oblique (major) fissure.
(b) Right pectoralis minor muscle.
(c) Right subclavian vein. This is dense on this image as it contains the intravenously administered contrast.
(d) Right subclavian artery.
(e) Horizontal (minor) fissure. The horizontal fissure bulges so that there is a convex upper border.

The horizontal fissure is higher medially than laterally and higher posteriorly than anteriorly. It is only present in the right lung since the left lung lacks a middle lobe. It normally extends from the oblique fissure at the level of the fourth rib.

6.17 Lateral C-spine radiograph

(a) Gas in vocal cord.
(b) Base of tongue.

(c) Hyoid bone.
(d) Styloid process.
(e) Anterior tubercle of transverse process of C5.

6.18 Lateral radiograph right wrist

(a) Trapezium.
(b) Lunate.
(c) Pisiform.
(d) Scaphoid.
(e) Ulnar styloid.

6.19 Sagittal T2-weighted MR pelvis (female)

(a) Pubic bone.
(b) Bladder.
(c) Endometrium.
(d) Rectus abdominus muscle.
(e) Junctional zone between myometrium and endometrium.

On T2-weighted images the endometrium is of high signal. The junctional zone is of low signal and the myometrium of intermediate signal.

6.20 Axial enhanced CT abdomen

(a) Duodenum – third part.
(b) Left anterior renal fascia.
(c) Left lateral conal fascia.
(d) Right posterior renal fascia.
(e) Retro-aortic left renal vein. A retro-aortic left renal vein is seen in about 2% of the population. In some situations the vein is posterior to the artery at the renal hilum. The anomalous vein may receive tributaries from the lumbar veins and can be associated with a higher incidence of left-sided varicoceles in males.

A circumaortic left renal vein occurs in about 8% of cases. There are two left renal veins – the superior component receives blood from the left adrenal vein and is anterior to the aorta. The inferior component is posterior to the aorta and receives blood from the gonadal vein. It is important in pre-operative planning of nephrectomy and in misdiagnosing lymphadenopathy.

Examination 7: Questions

Case 7.1

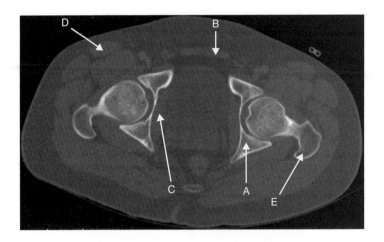

	QUESTION	WRITE YOUR ANSWER HERE
(a)	Name the structure labelled A.	
(b)	Name the structure labelled B.	
(c)	Name the structure labelled C.	
(d)	Name the structure labelled D.	
(e)	Name the structure labelled E.	

Case 7.2

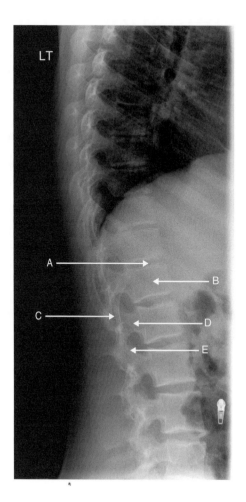

	QUESTION	WRITE YOUR ANSWER HERE
(a)	Name the structure labelled A.	
(b)	Name the structure labelled B.	
(c)	Name the structure labelled C.	
(d)	Name the structure labelled D.	
(e)	Name the structure labelled E.	

Case 7.3

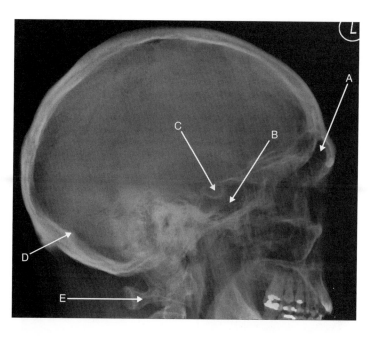

	QUESTION	WRITE YOUR ANSWER HERE
(a)	Name the structure labelled A.	
(b)	Name the structure labelled B.	
(c)	Name the structure labelled C.	
(d)	Name the structure labelled D.	
(e)	Name the structure labelled E.	

Case 7.4

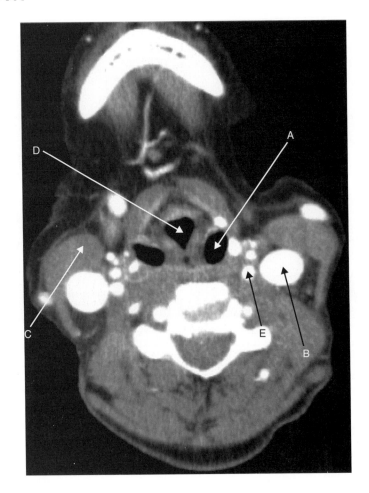

	QUESTION	WRITE YOUR ANSWER HERE
(a)	Name the structure labelled A.	
(b)	Name the structure labelled B.	
(c)	Name the structure labelled C.	
(d)	Name the structure labelled D.	
(e)	Name the structure labelled E.	

Case 7.5

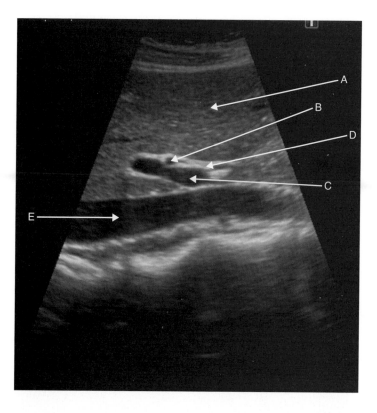

	QUESTION	WRITE YOUR ANSWER HERE
(a)	Name the structure labelled A.	
(b)	Name the structure labelled B.	
(c)	Name the structure labelled C.	
(d)	Name the structure labelled D.	
(e)	Name the structure labelled E.	

Case 7.6

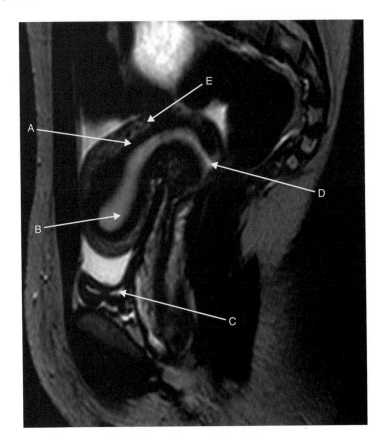

	QUESTION	WRITE YOUR ANSWER HERE
(a)	Name the structure labelled A.	
(b)	Name the structure labelled B.	
(c)	Name the structure labelled C.	
(d)	Name the structure labelled D.	
(e)	Name the structure labelled E.	

Case 7.7

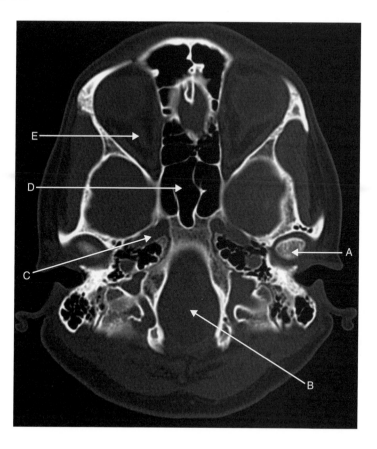

	QUESTION	WRITE YOUR ANSWER HERE
(a)	Name the structure labelled A.	
(b)	Name the structure labelled B.	
(c)	Name the structure labelled C.	
(d)	Name the structure labelled D.	
(e)	Name the structure labelled E.	

Case 7.8

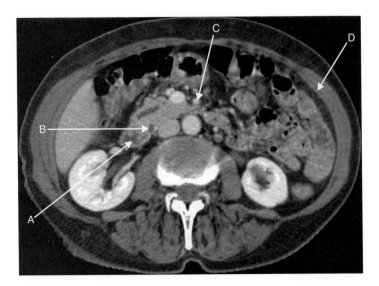

Image courtesy of Dr S. Sukumar, Wythenshawe Hospital, Manchester.

	QUESTION	WRITE YOUR ANSWER HERE
(a)	Name the structure labelled A	
(b)	Name the structure labelled B	
(c)	Name the structure labelled C	
(d)	Name the structure labelled D	
(e)	Which normal variant is present on this image?	

Case 7.9

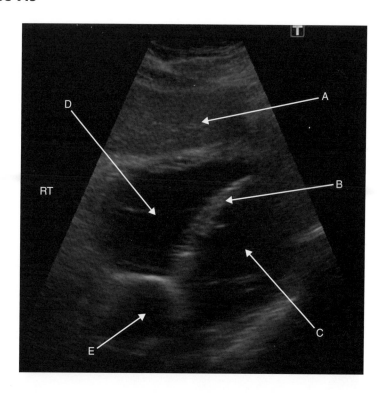

	QUESTION	WRITE YOUR ANSWER HERE
(a)	Name the structure labelled A.	
(b)	Name the structure labelled B.	
(c)	Name the structure labelled C.	
(d)	Name the structure labelled D.	
(e)	Name the structure labelled E.	

Case 7.10

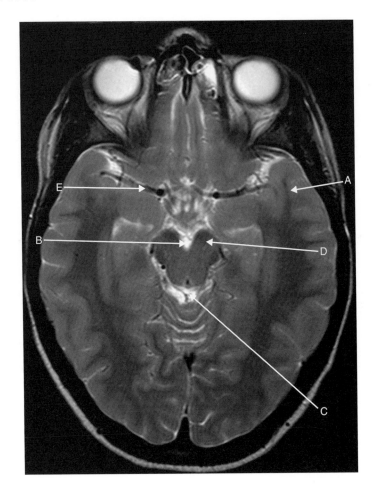

	QUESTION	WRITE YOUR ANSWER HERE
(a)	Name the structure labelled A.	
(b)	Name the structure labelled B.	
(c)	Name the structure labelled C.	
(d)	Name the structure labelled D.	
(e)	Name the structure labelled E.	

Case 7.11

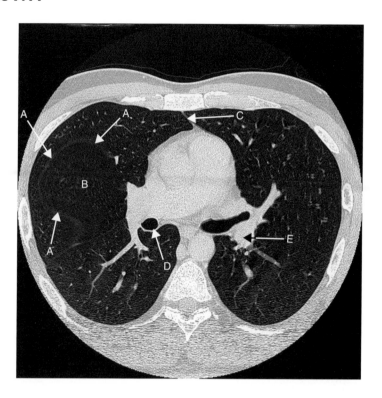

	QUESTION	WRITE YOUR ANSWER HERE
(a)	Name the structure labelled A.	
(b)	Name the structure labelled B.	
(c)	Name the structure labelled C.	
(d)	Name the structure labelled D.	
(e)	Name the structure labelled E.	

Case 7.12

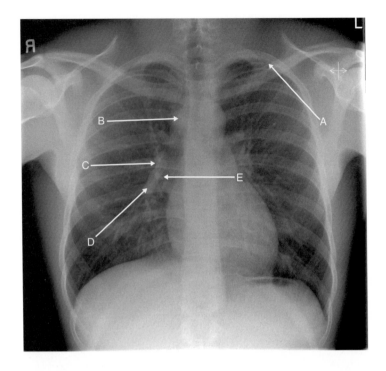

	QUESTION	WRITE YOUR ANSWER HERE
(a)	Name the structure labelled A.	
(b)	Name the structure labelled B.	
(c)	Name the structure labelled C.	
(d)	Name the structure labelled D.	
(e)	Name the structure labelled E.	

Case 7.13

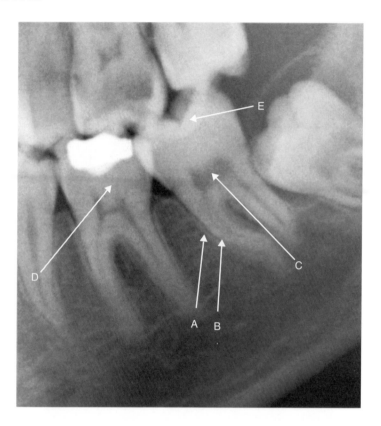

	QUESTION	WRITE YOUR ANSWER HERE
(a)	Name the structure labelled A.	
(b)	Name the structure labelled B.	
(c)	Name the structure labelled C.	
(d)	Name the structure labelled D.	
(e)	Name the structure labelled E.	

Case 7.14

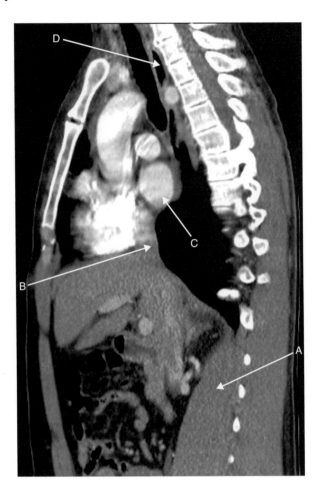

	QUESTION	WRITE YOUR ANSWER HERE
(a)	Name the structure labelled A.	
(b)	Name the structure labelled B.	
(c)	Name the structure labelled C.	
(d)	Name the structure labelled D.	
(e)	Which normal variant is present on this image?	

Case 7.15

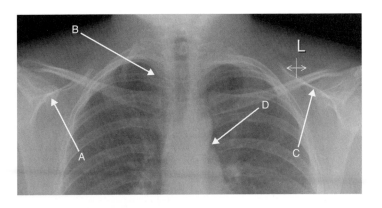

	QUESTION	WRITE YOUR ANSWER HERE
(a)	Name the structure labelled A.	
(b)	Name the structure labelled B.	
(c)	Name the structure labelled C.	
(d)	Name the structure labelled D.	
(e)	Which normal variant is present on this image?	

Case 7.16

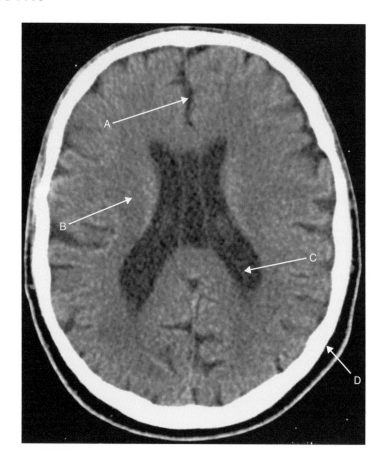

	QUESTION	WRITE YOUR ANSWER HERE
(a)	Name the structure labelled A.	
(b)	Name the structure labelled B.	
(c)	Name the structure labelled C.	
(d)	Name the structure labelled D.	
(e)	Which normal variant is present on this image?	

Case 7.17

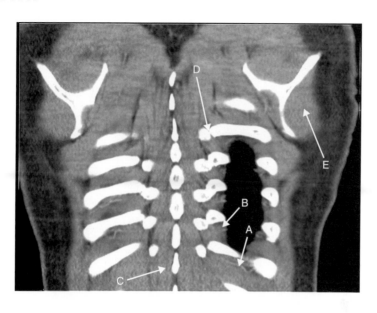

	QUESTION	WRITE YOUR ANSWER HERE
(a)	Name the structure labelled A.	
(b)	Name the structure labelled B.	
(c)	Name the structure labelled C.	
(d)	Name the structure labelled D.	
(e)	Name the structure labelled E.	

Case 7.18

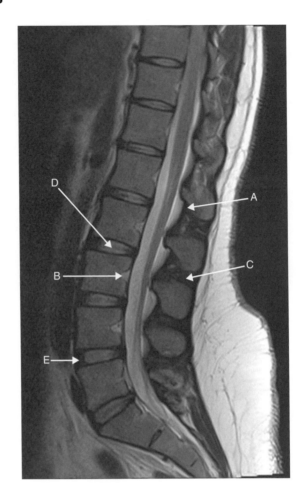

	QUESTION	WRITE YOUR ANSWER HERE
(a)	Name the structure labelled A.	
(b)	Name the structure labelled B.	
(c)	Name the structure labelled C.	
(d)	Name the structure labelled D.	
(e)	Name the structure labelled E.	

Case 7.19

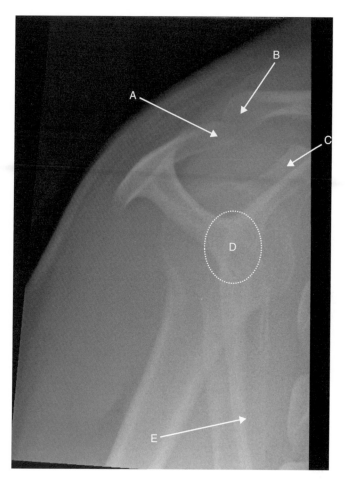

	QUESTION	WRITE YOUR ANSWER HERE
(a)	Name the structure labelled A.	
(b)	Name the structure labelled B.	
(c)	Name the structure labelled C.	
(d)	Name the structure labelled D.	
(e)	Name the structure labelled E.	

Case 7.20

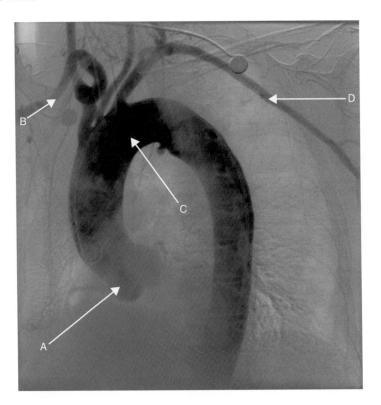

	QUESTION	WRITE YOUR ANSWER HERE
(a)	Name the structure labelled A.	
(b)	Name the structure labelled B.	
(c)	Name the structure labelled C.	
(d)	Name the structure labelled D.	
(e)	Which normal variant is present on this image?	

Examination 7: Answers

7.1 Axial CT pelvis (bone windows)

(a) Posterior column of the left acetabulum. The posterior and anterior columns of acetabulum provide the dominant load-bearing support of the hip joint. It is important to evaluate the integrity of the acetabular columns in the setting of pelvic trauma as fracture involvement of these structures is integral to all classification systems of acetabular fractures.

(b) Left rectus abdominis muscle. This is a strap-like muscle encased in a fascial sheath. It inserts onto the anterior surface of the pubic symphysis and has an aponeurosis which is continuous with that of the gracilis and adductor longus muscles.

(c) Right obturator internus. This arises from the internal surface of the medial acetabulum and inserts on the greater trochanter of the femur. Its action is to produce external rotation of the hip.

(d) Right sartorius muscle. This arises from the anterior superior iliac spine. It has a long muscle belly directed distally and medially spanning the hip and knee joints with an insertion on the antero-medial aspect of the tibia as one of the pes anseurinus tendon group.

(e) Greater trochanter of the left femur.

7.2 Lateral radiograph thoracolumbar spine

(a) T11/T12 disc space.
(b) T12 vertebral body.
(c) Twelfth rib.
(d) L1 pedicle.
(e) L1/L2 facet joint.

The interpedicular distance should increase to a maximum at the L5 level.
  Pedicular destruction is most common in metastatic disease.
  Irregularity of the endplates with loss of disc height is often seen in discitis.
  Less than 10 degrees of scoliosis is within normal limits.
  The lateral film demonstrates the depth of the posterior costophrenic angle with the lungs reaching the T12 level.

7.3 Lateral skull radiograph

(a) Frontal sinus.
(b) Sphenoid sinus.
(c) Pituitary fossa.
(d) Internal occipital protuberance.
(e) Posterior arch of C2.

Skull radiographs are no longer performed in trauma cases due to the poor sensitivity for intracerebral injury and the widespread availability of CT scans.

7.4 Axial enhanced CT neck

(a) Air in the left piriform fossa. This is part of the hypopharynx.

(b) Left internal jugular vein. The anterior branch of the retromandibular vein joins the facial vein to form the internal jugular vein.

(c) Right sternocleidomastoid muscle. The superior attachment is the mastoid process of the temporal bone. The inferior attachments are to the manubrium and the clavicle.

(d) Air in the supraglottic larynx. The supraglottic larynx consists of the false cords and aryepiglottic folds.

(e) Left internal carotid artery. This gives off two small branches in the petrous region – the caroticotympanic artery to the ear drum and the pterygoid artery to the pterygoid canal and plate. There are further small branches which come off in the cavernous region.

7.5 Ultrasound liver: oblique image through the porta hepatis

(a) Left lobe of the liver. The liver is typically a homogeneous mid-grey organ with echogenicity slightly increased when compared to cortex of right kidney.

(b) Hepatic artery. Generally crosses the anterior aspect of the portal vein with the common duct anterior to this. A common variant is the artery lying anterior to the common duct.

(c) Portal vein. This enters the liver and is encased by hyperechoic, fibrous walls of the portal tracts.

(d) Common bile duct. This is best seen with the patient supine in a right anterior oblique position. Typically measures approximately 6 mm or less. However, it is age dependent and can be 8–9 mm in the elderly.

(e) Inferior vena cava (IVC). The three hepatic veins drain into the IVC just inferior to the diaphragm. The attachment helps hold the liver in position. The IVC runs posteriorly to the liver before passing through the caval opening in the diaphragm at T8 level.

7.6 Sagittal T2-weighted MR female pelvis

(a) Junctional zone of uterus.

(b) Endometrial cavity.

(c) Urinary bladder.

(d) External os of uterus.

(e) Myometrium of uterus.

Ultrasound, both transabdominal and transvaginal, and MRI are used to assess the female pelvis. MRI has superior soft tissue contrast, and can delineate anatomy very clearly. On T2 sequences the endometrium, endocervical canal and vaginal canal are of high signal. The inner zone of the myometrium is of low signal and known as the junctional zone. This is histologically similar to the remainder of the myometrium. The outer myometrium is of intermediate signal. There is high signal pelvic fluid.

T1-weighted images of the uterus and ovaries show intermediate signal with poor contrast.

Fibroids (leiomyoma) are the most common tumour of the uterus, found in 25% of females >35 years. They arise from smooth muscle cells and can be well visualized on MRI. They are typically seen as low signal lesions relative to the remainder of the uterus on T2-weighted images and isointense to the uterus on T1-weighted images.

7.7 Axial CT skull base (bone windows)

(a) Left head (condyle) of mandible.

(b) Foramen magnum. With raised intracranial pressure from any aetiology (traumatic, neoplastic, ischaemic) the cerebellar tonsils can descend through the foramen magnum which is known as tonsillar herniation. This causes compression of the cardiac and respiratory centres within the brainstem and thereby death. This is best appreciated on sagittal MR though can be suspected on CT. Other possible brain herniations include:

    1. transtentorial (or uncal) herniation where the medial aspect of the temporal lobe (uncus) herniates inferior to the tentorium cerebelli

    2. subfalcine herniation where a frontal lobe crosses the midline and passes beneath the falx cerebri (midline shift).

(c) Right carotid canal. Part of the petrous apex of the temporal bone.

(d) Sphenoid sinus. There are varying degrees of pneumatization of the sphenoid sinus in individuals. The sphenoid sinuses drain into the sphenoethmoidal recesses, either side of the nasal septum.

(e) Right optic nerve.

7.8 Axial enhanced abdominal CT

(a) Second part of duodenum.

(b) Common bile duct (CBD).

(c) Superior mesenteric artery.

(d) Left internal oblique muscle.

(e) Pancreas divisum. This anomaly is present in up to 14% of the population (in autopsy series). Normally the shorter ventral duct (Wirsung), which drains the head of the pancreas, joins the CBD (labelled B) to drain via the major papilla into the duodenum. There is failure of fusion of the ventral duct with the main dorsal pancreatic duct (Santorini), which drain the body of the pancreas. The dorsal duct drains into the duodenum via the minor papilla. There is an unproven suggestion that this anomaly predisposes to pancreatitis.

7.9 Echocardiogram

(a) Left lobe of the liver.

(b) Interventricular septum (IVS). This is composed of muscular and membranous parts. Due to the high blood pressure in the left ventricle the muscular part of the IVS forms the majority of the septum.

(c) Left ventricle. This forms the apex and nearly all the left surface of the heart.

(d) Right ventricle. This forms the majority of the anterior surface of the heart.

(e) Left atrium. This forms most of the base of the heart. Four pulmonary veins enter its smooth posterior wall.

7.10 Axial T2-weighted MR brain

(a) Left temporal lobe.

(b) Interpedicular cistern.

(c) Quadrigeminal cistern.

(d) Left cerebral peduncle.

(e) Right middle cerebral artery (MCA). The arrow points at the horizontal or M1 segment of the MCA. This gives off a number of lenticulostriate arteries which perfuse the lateral basal ganglia. At the insula, the artery turns into the Sylvian fissure (M2 segment) giving off a number of insular branches. The branches emerge form the lateral aspect of the Sylvian fissure extending anteriorly and posteriorly over the frontal, parietal and temporal lobes (M3 segment).

In acute stroke thrombus can be seen within the MCA. On CT, this is called the hyperdense MCA sign if the thrombus is in the M1 segment, and if it is in the M2 segment as the hyperdense MCA dot sign.

7.11 Axial CT thorax (bone windows)

(a) Minor or horizontal fissure.
(b) Right middle lobe.
(c) Anterior junction line.
(d) Posterior wall of bronchus intermedius.
(e) Left lower lobe pulmonary artery.

HRCT has sufficient resolution to depict the fissures as thin lines. On conventional non-thin slice CT, low attenuation areas of avascularity represent the fissures.
   The horizontal fissure on axial slices encircles the right middle lobe. This is because the horizontal fissure is convex superiorly.

7.12 PA chest radiograph

(a) Companion shadow of left clavicle.
(b) Azygos vein.
(c) Right hilar point.
(d) Right interlobar pulmonary artery.
(e) Bronchus intermedius. The pulmonary arteries are always located alongside bronchi. In the case of bronchus intermedius, it lies adjacent to the interlobar artery.

7.13 Bitewing x-ray

(a) Lamina dura. This is a dense white line of bone surrounding the root of each tooth.
(b) Periodontal ligament. This is the radiolucent line around the neck and root of the tooth.
(c) Pulp chamber. The pulp canals extend inferiorly from this and transmit nerves and vessels from the supporting bone.
(d) Dentine.
(e) Enamel. This is the densest material in the body.

7.14 Sagittal enhanced CT thorax and abdomen

(a) Right psoas muscle. (Right side because the aortic root can be seen. Plus see answer (e).)
(b) Inferior vena cava.
(c) Left atrium.
(d) Oesophagus.
(e) Aberrant right subclavian artery. The aberrant right subclavian artery arises from the aorta distal to the left subclavian artery, traverses behind the oesophagus to supply the right arm. It will produce a posterior impression on the oesophagus at barium swallow.

7.15 PA chest radiograph

(a) Coracoid process of the right scapula.
(b) Right transverse process of T3.
(c) Spine of left scapula.
(d) Aorto-pulmonary window.
(e) Right cervical rib. A cervical rib articulates with a transverse process which is orientated in a downwards direction unlike thoracic ribs, which articulate with an upwardly orientated transverse process. They may cause vascular and neural compression leading to symptoms in the upper limb.

7.16 Axial unenhanced brain CT

(a) Falx cerebri.
(b) Left corona radiata.
(c) Posterior horn of the left lateral ventricle.
(d) Left parietal bone.
(e) Cavum vergae. This is a normal variant similar to cavum septum pellucidum except in this case the separation of the septum pellucidum leaflets extends back to the splenium of the corpus callosum.

7.17 Coronal enhanced thorax CT

(a) Left intercostal artery.
(b) Left intercostal vein.
(c) Left erector spinae muscle.
(d) Left costotransverse joint.
(e) Left infraspinatus muscle.

The intercostal neurovascular bundle is exposed posteriorly and has no protection from the bony intercostal groove. This is very different to the situation that exists in the antero-lateral chest wall where the neurovascular bundle is protected by the subcostal groove. The neurovascular bundle is situated between the internal and innermost intercostal muscles. The lack of protection posteriorly makes chest drain insertion and percutaneous intrathoracic biopsy procedures particularly hazardous with resulting haemothoraces as the most serious complication if there is arterial puncture. Therefore, great care must be taken when accessing the thorax via a posterior approach. Avoidance of this route is preferable but if access must be made at this site, a caudal tilt to the needle so that it glances the superior aspect of the rib below is advisable in order to reduce the risk of arterial puncture.

7.18 Sagittal T2-weighted MR lumbar spine

(a) Ligamentum flavum.
(b) Basivertebral vein.
(c) Interspinous ligament.
(d) Nucleus pulposus of L2/L3 disc
(e) Annulus fibrosis of L4/L5 disc.

7.19 Y-view right shoulder radiograph

(a) Acromion.
(b) Clavicle.

(c) Coracoid process.
(d) Glenoid.
(e) Lateral scapular border.

7.20 Arch aortogram

(a) Anterior aortic cusp (or sinus of Valsalva). The right coronary artery arises from here. The left coronary artery arises from the left posterior sinus.
(b) Right subclavian artery.
(c) Aortic arch. The aortic arch is defined as the aorta from the right brachiocephalic artery to the attachment of the ligamentum arteriosum. It can be further subdivided into proximal arch (right brachiocephalic artery to left subclavian artery (LSA)) and distal (LSA to attachment of ligament arteriosum). The distal arch is sometimes referred to as the isthmus or 'bridge' and may be narrower than the proximal descending aorta. The isthmus represents the weakest part of the arch and is prone to transection, intimal laceration and false aneurysm formation in decelerating road traffic accidents.
(d) Left axillary artery.
(e) Ductus diverticulum ('ductus bump'). This is a fusiform dilatation along the ventro-medial aspect of the descending aorta adjacent to the ligamentum arteriosum. It is present in up to 9% of adults. Its appearances are sometimes confounding in blunt trauma as it can be confused with a false aneurysm. This point on the aorta is a transition between the fixed descending aorta and mobile aortic arch, and therefore represents a site where transection and focal aneurysm can occur.

Examination 8: Questions

Case 8.1

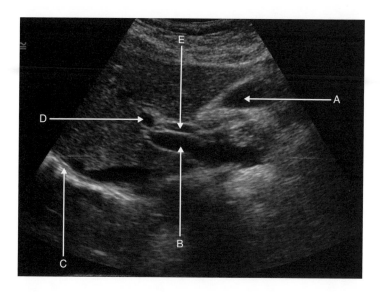

	QUESTION	WRITE YOUR ANSWER HERE
(a)	Name the structure labelled A.	
(b)	Name the structure labelled B.	
(c)	Name the structure labelled C.	
(d)	Name the structure labelled D.	
(e)	Name the structure labelled E.	

Case 8.2

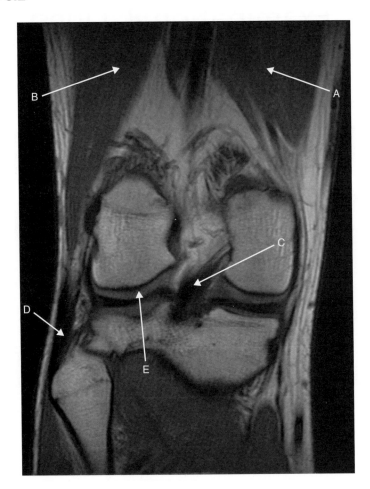

	QUESTION	WRITE YOUR ANSWER HERE
(a)	Name the structure labelled A.	
(b)	Name the structure labelled B.	
(c)	Name the structure labelled C.	
(d)	Name the structure labelled D.	
(e)	Name the structure labelled E.	

Case 8.3

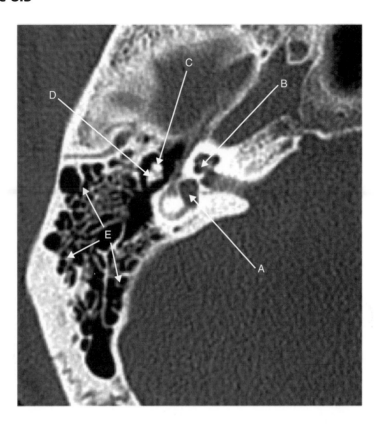

	QUESTION	WRITE YOUR ANSWER HERE
(a)	Name the structure labelled A.	
(b)	Name the structure labelled B.	
(c)	Name the structure labelled C.	
(d)	Name the structure labelled D.	
(e)	Name the structure labelled E.	

Case 8.4

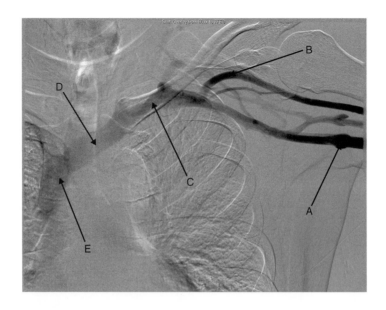

	QUESTION	WRITE YOUR ANSWER HERE
(a)	Name the structure labelled A.	
(b)	Name the structure labelled B.	
(c)	Name the structure labelled C.	
(d)	Name the structure labelled D.	
(e)	Name the structure labelled E.	

Case 8.5

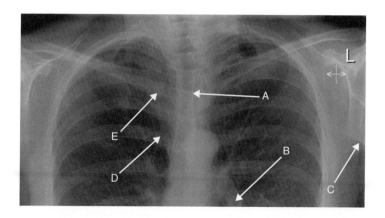

	QUESTION	WRITE YOUR ANSWER HERE
(a)	Name the structure labelled A.	
(b)	Name the structure labelled B.	
(c)	Name the structure labelled C.	
(d)	Name the structure labelled D.	
(e)	Name the structure labelled E.	

Case 8.6

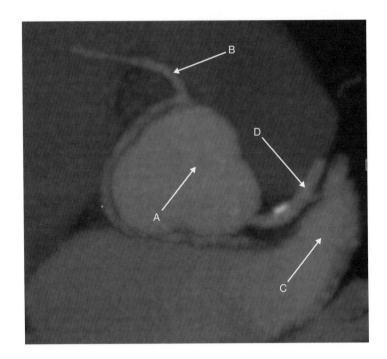

	QUESTION	WRITE YOUR ANSWER HERE
(a)	Name the structure labelled A.	
(b)	Name the structure labelled B.	
(c)	Name the structure labelled C.	
(d)	Name the structure labelled D.	
(e)	Which normal variant is present on this image?	

Case 8.7

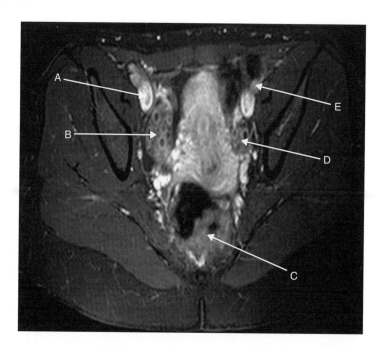

	QUESTION	WRITE YOUR ANSWER HERE
(a)	Name the structure labelled A.	
(b)	Name the structure labelled B.	
(c)	Name the structure labelled C.	
(d)	Name the structure labelled D.	
(e)	Name the structure labelled E.	

Case 8.8

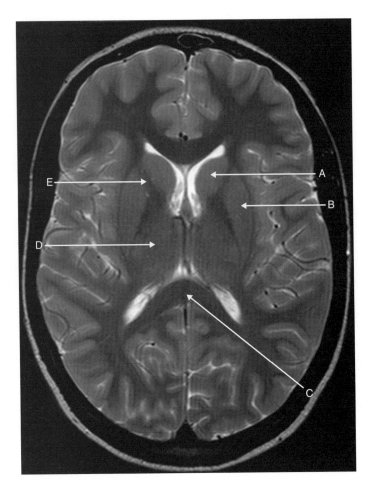

	QUESTION	WRITE YOUR ANSWER HERE
(a)	Name the structure labelled A.	
(b)	Name the structure labelled B.	
(c)	Name the structure labelled C.	
(d)	Name the structure labelled D.	
(e)	Name the structure labelled E.	

Case 8.9

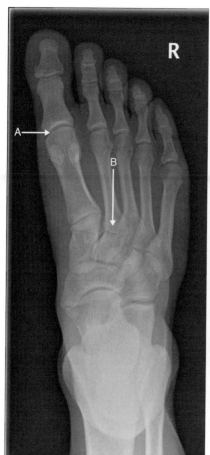 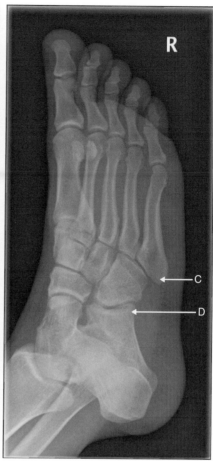

	QUESTION	WRITE YOUR ANSWER HERE
(a)	Name the structure labelled A.	
(b)	Name the structure labelled B.	
(c)	Name the structure labelled C.	
(d)	Name the structure labelled D.	
(e)	Which normal variant is present on this image?	

Case 8.10

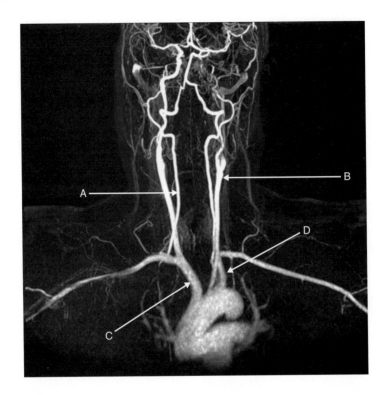

	QUESTION	WRITE YOUR ANSWER HERE
(a)	Name the structure labelled A.	
(b)	Name the structure labelled B.	
(c)	Name the structure labelled C.	
(d)	Name the structure labelled D.	
(e)	Which normal variant is present on this image?	

Case 8.11

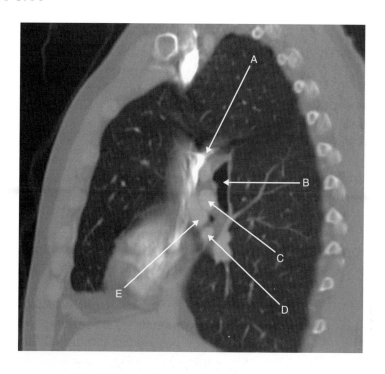

	QUESTION	WRITE YOUR ANSWER HERE
(a)	Name the structure labelled A.	
(b)	Name the structure labelled B.	
(c)	Name the structure labelled C.	
(d)	Name the structure labelled D.	
(e)	Name the structure labelled E.	

Case 8.12

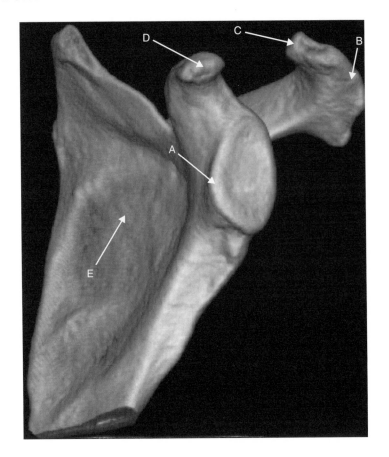

	QUESTION	WRITE YOUR ANSWER HERE
(a)	Name the structure labelled A.	
(b)	Name the structure labelled B.	
(c)	Name the structure which attaches to the point labelled C.	
(d)	Name the structure labelled D.	
(e)	Name the structure which attaches to the fossa labelled E.	

Case 8.13

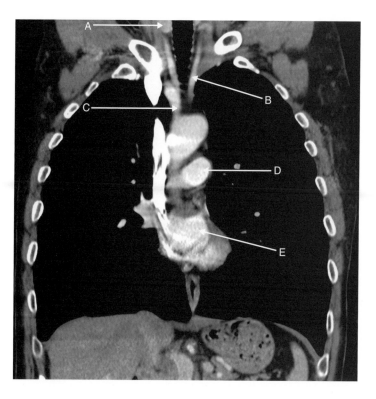

	QUESTION	WRITE YOUR ANSWER HERE
(a)	Name the structure labelled A.	
(b)	Name the structure labelled B.	
(c)	Name the structure labelled C.	
(d)	Name the structure labelled D.	
(e)	Name the structure labelled E.	

Case 8.14

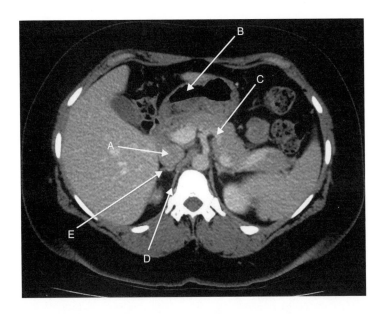

	QUESTION	WRITE YOUR ANSWER HERE
(a)	Name the structure labelled A.	
(b)	Name the structure labelled B.	
(c)	Name the structure labelled C.	
(d)	Name the structure labelled D.	
(e)	Name the structure labelled E.	

Case 8.15

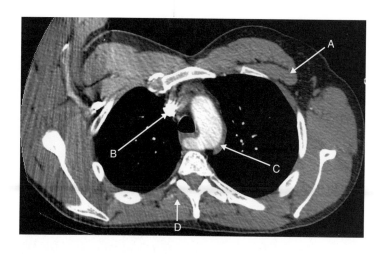

	QUESTION	WRITE YOUR ANSWER HERE
(a)	Name the structure labelled A.	
(b)	Name the structure labelled B.	
(c)	Name the structure labelled C.	
(d)	Name the structure labelled D.	
(e)	Which normal variant is present on this image?	

Case 8.16

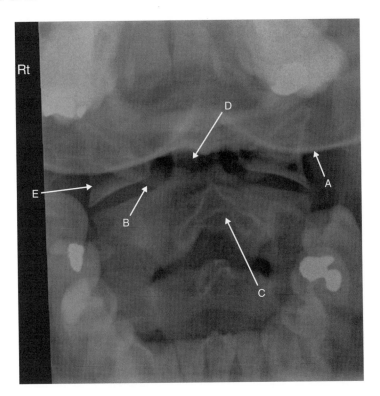

	QUESTION	WRITE YOUR ANSWER HERE
(a)	Name the structure labelled A.	
(b)	Name the structure labelled B.	
(c)	Name the structure labelled C.	
(d)	Name the structure labelled D.	
(e)	Name the structure labelled E.	

Case 8.17

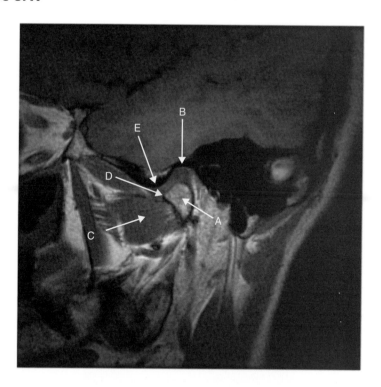

	QUESTION	WRITE YOUR ANSWER HERE
(a)	Name the structure labelled A.	
(b)	Name the structure labelled B.	
(c)	Name the structure labelled C.	
(d)	Name the structure labelled D.	
(e)	Name the structure labelled E.	

Case 8.18

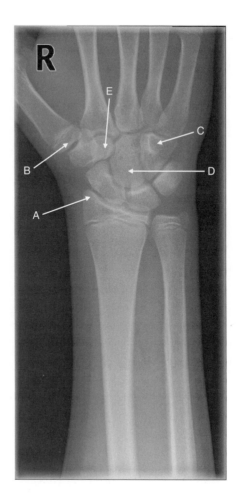

	QUESTION	WRITE YOUR ANSWER HERE
(a)	Name the structure labelled A.	
(b)	Name the structure labelled B.	
(c)	Name the structure labelled C.	
(d)	Name the structure labelled D.	
(e)	Name the structure labelled E.	

Case 8.19

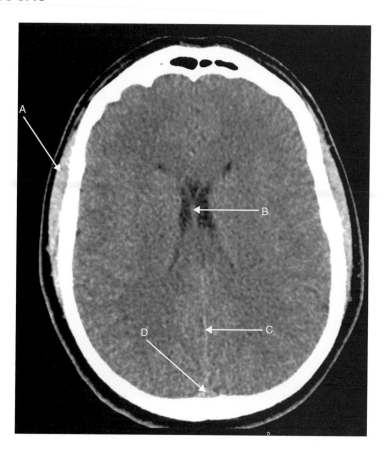

	QUESTION	WRITE YOUR ANSWER HERE
(a)	Name the structure labelled A.	
(b)	Name the structure labelled B.	
(c)	Name the structure labelled C.	
(d)	Name the structure labelled D.	
(e)	Which normal variant is present on this image?	

Case 8.20

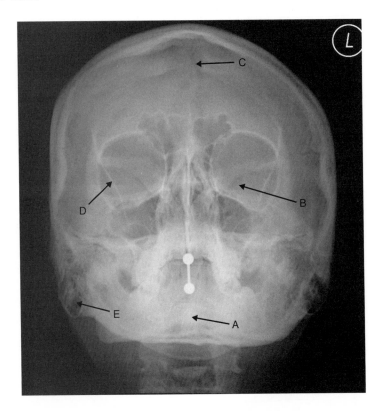

	QUESTION	WRITE YOUR ANSWER HERE
(a)	Name the structure labelled A.	
(b)	Name the structure labelled B.	
(c)	Name the structure labelled C.	
(d)	Name the structure labelled D.	
(e)	Name the structure labelled E.	

Examination 8: Answers

8.1 Transverse ultrasound through the porta hepatis

(a) Gallbladder. The gallbladder stores about 50 ml of bile. Its blood supply is from the cystic artery, a branch of the right hepatic artery. It drains into segment 5 of the liver where it also receives a collateral blood supply. There are folds in the mucous membrane of the cystic duct (spiral valve of Heister) which together with underlying smooth muscle serve to regulate the flow of bile.

(b) Portal vein. It forms at the confluence of the splenic and superior mesenteric vein at L1/L2 level, posterior to the neck of the pancreas.

   The portal vein provides 75% of the liver's inflow with the common hepatic artery supplying the remainder. Of note however, if there is a malignancy within the liver (primary or secondary) its blood supply is invariably arterial in origin.

(c) Right hemidiaphragm. The lung above the diaphragm is not seen as air conducts the ultrasound poorly. If there is a plural effusion however, it will be apparent in this region.

(d) Common hepatic artery. The region of the liver containing the common hepatic artery, common hepatic duct and portal vein is known as the porta hepatis.

(e) Common bile duct. This becomes the common bile duct (CBD) after the confluence with the cystic duct. The normal diameter of the CBD is variable but more than 8 mm can be pathological, though it dilates with increasing age. Generally 1 mm per decade gives a useful approximation.

8.2 Coronal T1-weighted MR right knee

(a) Vastus medialis muscle.

(b) Vastus lateralis muscle.

(c) Anterior cruciate ligament. There is an aide memoire for remembering the orientation of the cruciate ligaments.

   The anterior cruciate ligament is extrasynovial, intracapsular and arises from the intercondylar notch in the tibia and rises towards the anterior aspect of the lateral femoral condyle. Anterior – Backwards, Upwards and Laterally (ABUL).

   The posterior cruciate ligament is intrasynovial, extracapsular and arises from the posterior tibial plateau and rises towards the posterior aspect of the medial femoral condyle. Posterior – Upwards, Medially and Forwards (PUMF).

(d) Conjoined tendon. The conjoined tendon is the combination of the lateral collateral ligament and biceps femoris tendon inserting onto the fibular head. The lateral stabilizing ligaments comprise:

   Superficial layer – iliotibial band anteriorly merging with the biceps femoris tendon posteriorly

   Intermediate layer – postero-lateral collateral ligament

   Deep layer – popliteus tendon.

(e) Hyaline cartilage of lateral femoral condyle.

8.3 HRCT right inner ear

(a) Right vestibule. This communicates posteriorly with the three semicircular canals and anteriorly with the cochlear.

(b) Right cochlear. This contains the cell bodies of the cochlear nerve within the modiolus.

(c) Right head of malleus. The handle of the malleus is attached to the tympanic membrane whilst the head articulates with the body of the incus.

(d) Right body of incus. The body of the incus articulates with the malleus at the incudomallear joint. The long process of the incus articulates with the head of the stapes.

(e) Right mastoid air cells. These communicate with the attic via the aditus ad antrum.

8.4 Venogram left upper limb

(a) Valve in left basilic vein.

(b) Left cephalic vein. The cephalic vein, in the forearm and at the elbow, is the primary vein utilized in fashioning arteriovenous fistulae (AVF) for haemodialysis. The arrowed segment is known as the terminal arch and is notorious for developing stenoses secondary to distal AVF.

(c) Left subclavian vein. This is a continuation of the axillary vein at the outer border of the first rib and combines with the jugular vein at the sternal end of the clavicle.

(d) Left brachiocephalic vein.

(e) Superior vena cava (SVC).

8.5 PA chest radiograph centred over the upper mediastinum

(a) Posterior junction line. The posterior junction line is seen in about 30% of PA chest radiographs and is formed when the x-ray beam is tangential to the apposition of the postero-medial portion of both upper lobes posteriorly. On the PA radiograph it runs from above the clavicles to the arch of the aorta and is projected through the trachea. The line comprises four layers – two parietal and two visceral pleural layers. The line may become a stripe if there is a significant amount of mediastinal fat in between the two lungs.

Abnormal bulging of this line suggests mass lesions of the oesophagus, lymphadenopathy or neurogenic masses.

(b) Left main pulmonary artery. The left main pulmonary artery is more cranial in position than the right main pulmonary artery since it is superior to the left main bronchus just prior to its bifurcation.

(c) Left axillary fold.

(d) Right lateral border of the sternum.

(e) Right sternoclavicular joint. The sternoclavicular joint is a synovial joint separated by a flat articular disc. There are four strong ligaments (anterior and posterior sternoclavicular, interclavicular and costoclavicular) and a strong fibrous capsule. As a result trauma to the joint rarely causes disruption but instead is associated with clavicular fracture.

8.6 Coronary CT

(a) Aortic root.

(b) Right coronary artery (RCA).

(c) Left atrial appendage.

(d) Left anterior descending artery.

(e) Aberrant left circumflex artery (LCX). In this case the anomalous LCX arises from the right sinus of Valsalva and shares a common origin with the RCA. It then runs behind the aortic root to reach the left atrioventricular groove and supply the lateral left ventricular wall. The anomalous LCX may have a separate origin from the RCA in the right sinus of Valsalva.

Anomalous coronary arteries are seen in 0.6–1.5% of catheter angiograms and an anomalous LCX is the commonest normal variant of coronary artery anatomy. CT coronary angiography is the examination of choice if anomalous coronary artery anatomy is suspected, and it is essential to know the variant anatomy if percutaneous coronary intervention or aortic root surgery is being considered.

8.7 Axial T2-weighted MR pelvis (female)

(a) Right femoral vein.
(b) Right ovary.
(c) Rectum.
(d) Left ovary.
(e) Left femoral artery.

MRI is commonly used in assessing both the male and the female pelvis. Fat saturation techniques can enable the pelvic organs to be well visualized. Ovarian cysts can be seen, which are often small and multiple in pre-menopausal females.

8.8 Axial T2-weighted MR image of the brain

(a) Left caudate nucleus.
(b) Left lentiform nucleus. This consists of two components – the lateral putamen and medial globus pallidus.
   Together the lentiform and caudate nuclei are known as the corpus striatum. They are part of the extrapyramidal system of the motor system, involved in the coordination of reflexes and posture.
(c) Splenium of the corpus callosum. The corpus callosum connects both cerebral hemispheres. The splenium is the bulky posterior part, anterior to which lies the body, genu and rostrum respectively.
(d) Right thalamus.
(e) Anterior limb of the right internal capsule.

8.9 AP and oblique radiograph of the right foot

(a) First metatarso-phalangeal joint. A common place to look for primary osteoarthritis which results clinically in hallux rigidus. If rheumatoid arthritis affects this joint then the result is hallux valgus. Gout also has a predilection for this joint although is now rarely seen on imaging due to the efficacy of medical management.
(b) Base of the second metatarsal. This is held in place by a mortice made by the medial, middle and lateral cuneiform bones and is informally referred to as the Lisfranc joint. It is important to verify alignment on trauma films to rule out a midfoot (Lisfranc) dislocation:
  - On the AP view the medial margin of the base of the second metatarsal should align with the medial margin of the middle cuneiform.
  - On the oblique view the medial margin of the base of the third metatarsal should align with the medial margin of the lateral cunieform.

(c) Tuberosity of the fifth metatarsal. A common place of avulsion fractures due to inversion injuries. If the fracture line lies within the proximal diaphysis (distal to the joint line of the fourth tarsometatarsal joint), then this fracture is known as a Jones' fracture, which notoriously results in delayed or non-union. It is not an avulsion fracture. The Jones' fracture is named after Sir Robert Jones (1857–1933), Professor of Orthopaedic Surgery at Liverpool University.

(d) Calcaneum.

(e) Os tibiale externum. This can lie entirely separately within the tendon of tibialis posterior (type 1) or have a cartilaginous (type II) or osseous (type III) connection with the medial aspect of the navicular bone.

8.10 MRA carotids

(a) Right vertebral artery.

(b) Left common carotid artery. The left internal carotid artery just superior to this is seen to be occluded on this study.

(c) Brachiocephalic trunk (innominate artery).

(d) Left subclavian artery.

(e) Left vertebral artery arising directly from the arch of the aorta. This occurs in 6% of the population, with the most frequent location for its origin being between the left common carotid and subclavian arteries.

8.11 Sagittal CT chest

(a) Azygos vein.

(b) Bronchus intermedius.

(c) Right interlobar pulmonary artery. The right interlobar and upper lobe pulmonary arteries both lie *anterior* to bronchus intermedius. (On the left side the pulmonary artery lies *posterior* to the left main bronchus.)

(d) Right inferior pulmonary vein.

(e) Right superior pulmonary vein. The right pulmonary veins lie *anterior* to the pulmonary arteries.

8.12 3D volume rendering of the scapula

(a) Antero-inferior glenoid rim. This is an important region as it bears the attachment of the anterior band of the inferior glenohumeral ligament (AIGHL). This is the site of avulsion fracture sustained during anterior glenohumeral dislocation known as a bony Bankart lesion. The classic Bankart lesion refers to avulsion of the antero-inferior glenoid labrum along with the AIGHL and thus cannot be seen on radiographs.

(b) Acromion process. The deltoid origin is broad and curved and extends around the entire border of the acromion. Bony avulsion of the acromion is rare following trauma though enthesopathy at the deltoid origin is a common degenerative feature on radiographs.

(c) Coraco-acromial ligament (CAL). The CAL is a narrow but tough ligament that arises from the anterior tip of the acromial undersurface. Its origin may form a bony enthesophyte that has been implicated in the aetiology of supraspinatus tendon tears. The CAL is thought to contribute to the clinical condition of sub-acromial impingement and it is routinely divided during a sub-acromial decompression procedure.

(d) Coracoid process. The coracobrachialis is a long muscle that arises from the coracoid process and inserts distally on the antero-medial surface of the humeral diaphysis.

(e) Subscapularis. As its name suggests the subscapularis is a broad multi-pennate muscle that lies beneath the scapula. It becomes narrower laterally, as does the shape of the scapula, to form a broad tendon that inserts on the lesser tuberosity of the humerus which acts to internally rotate the shoulder.

8.13 Coronal contrast-enhanced CT chest

(a) Right thyroid lobe.
(b) Left common carotid artery.
(c) Brachiocephalic trunk.
(d) Left pulmonary artery.
(e) Left atrium.

8.14 Axial portal venous phase abdominal CT

(a) Inferior vena cava.
(b) Gastric antrum.
(c) Splenic artery.
(d) Crus of the right hemidiaphragm.
(e) Lateral limb of the right adrenal gland.

8.15 Axial arterial phase CT thorax

(a) Left pectoralis minor muscle.
(b) Superior vena cava.
(c) Left superior intercostal vein.
(d) Right erector spinae muscle.
(e) Aberrant right subclavian artery.

8.16 C-spine odontoid peg view

(a) Occipital bone.
(b) Anterior arch of the atlas (C1).
(c) Spinous process of C2.
(d) Dens (odontoid peg).
(e) Right lateral mass of C1.

8.17 Temporomandibular MRI

(a) Condylar head. The temporomandibular joint is a synovial joint between the condyle of the mandible and the articular fossa of the temporal bone.
(b) Articular fossa. The head of the mandible sits in the fossa at rest.
(c) Lateral pterygoid muscle. This attaches to the anterior band of the articular disc.
(d) Anterior band of the articular disc. The articular disc has an anterior and posterior band with a thin zone in the middle. The disc is attached to the joint capsule. The joint space is divided into upper and lower compartments by the disc.
(e) Articular eminence. The head of the condyle moves anteriorly against the eminence on jaw opening.

8.18 AP radiograph of paediatric wrist

(a) Radial styloid epiphysis.
(b) Base of thumb epiphysis.
(c) Hook of hamate.
(d) Capitate.
(e) Trapezoid.

8.19 Axial unenhanced CT brain

(a) Right temporalis muscle.
(b) Septum pellucidum.
(c) Falx cerebri.
(d) Superior sagittal sinus.
(e) Cavum septum pellucidum. Cavum septum pellucidum (CSP) is a potential space filled with cerebrospinal fluid that occurs between the leaflets of the septum pellucidum. It is limited posteriorly by the fornix, unlike cavum vergae, which extends as far back as the splenium of the corpus callosum. It is present in 100% of fetuses with approximately 85% fusing by 6 months.

8.20 AP radiograph facial bones

(a) Odontoid peg.
(b) Left superior orbital fissure.
(c) Sagittal suture.
(d) Right greater wing of sphenoid.
(e) Right mastoid process.